The Natural Hygiene Diet

The Natural Hygiene Diet

From the Editors of *Health Science* Magazine

American Natural Hygiene Society, Inc.

The Natural Hygiene Diet
First Edition 1999

American Natural Hygiene Society, Inc.
P.O. Box 30630, Tampa, FL 33630

Appreciation:
We want to thank everyone who has shared articles, personal experiences, and other expertise in *Health Science* magazine. It is from this body of knowledge and experience that *The Natural Hygiene Diet* was compiled.

Editors:
James Michael Lennon and Susan Taylor

Copy Editors:
Linda Grudnik and Terry Kennedy

ISBN 0-914532-44-8
Library of Congress Catalog Number: 98-74701

PRINTED IN THE UNITED STATES OF AMERICA

Printed on Recycled Paper

Special Thanks

The publication of this book was made possible by a grant from the James Hervey Johnson Charitable Educational Trust.

James Hervey Johnson (1901-1988) was an active member of the American Natural Hygiene Society. His legacy of commitment to Natural Hygiene spans the decades to the present day.

Mr. Johnson was active for many years and held office in the Society's local chapter in San Diego. In 1963, he was the chairman and host of the Society's ANHS International Natural Living Conference in his hometown of San Diego, Calif.

The American Natural Hygiene Society gratefully thanks the James Hervey Johnson Charitable Educational Trust, Kevin Munnelly, Trustee, for helping the Society spread Mr. Johnson's health views—Natural Hygiene, the science of health.

Publisher's Note

Nothing in this book is intended to constitute medical treatment or advice of any nature.This book describes a general approach to healthful eating that is well-documented in the scientific literature. However, since every person is unique, with individual needs and capacities, no dietary recommendations could ever meet the precise needs of every individual. Moreover, as every person responds differently to diet and lifestyle modification, it is strongly recommended that any person desiring to make dramatic diet or lifestyle changes consult with his or her physician.

Acknowledgements

We acknowledge our indebtedness to everyone who has contributed to *Health Science* magazine and to ANHS Conferences over the years, upon whose expertise, experience, and observations the information and opinions in this book have been based.

We would especially like to thank: Alec Burton, M.Sc., D.O., D.C., and Nejla Burton, D.O., D.C., of Australia; Alan Goldhamer, D.C., Jennifer Marano, D.C., Douglas Lisle, Ph.D., and Susan Smith Jones, Ph.D., of California; Ronald G. Cridland, M.D., and Philip Martin, D.C., of Canada; Keki Sidhwa, N.D., D.O., of England; Frank Sabatino, D.C., Ph.D., and Jeff Novick, R.D., L.D., of Florida; Paula Duvall of Indiana; Joel Fuhrman, M.D., of New Jersey; Joy Gross of New York; D.J. Scott, D.C., of Ohio; and Ralph C. Cinque, D.C., of Texas.

We also thank Drs. Gerald Benesh of California and William Esser of Florida, the two surviving ANHS co-founders, for their vision and support.

Special recognition must go to T. Colin Campbell, Ph.D., of Cornell University, whose "China Study" research has opened a new era in the study of human nutrition.

This project could not have reached fruition without the ongoing support of the ANHS Board of Directors: Mark A. Huberman, President; Mark Epstein, Vice President; Dorothy Brosious, Treasurer; Meg Friedrich, Secretary; David Aukamp, D.C.; Harold Hoffman; Dawn Kimble; Jean Oswald; Daniel Regan; Lauren Rosenstadt; and Elaine Schuler.

Finally, this book would not be the same without the insightful cartoons of Sidney Harris.

Dedication

We dedicate this book to the men and women who during the past 160 years have dedicated their lives to carrying the vital Natural Hygiene message of "health through healthful living" to people around the world. By their numerous efforts, large and small, these men and women have marked themselves as leaders of the great and noble work of building a healthier and happier world for everyone, everywhere.

Table of Contents

Introduction

Natural Hygiene is a timeless approach to health and happiness that has helped to transform the lives of countless thousands of people. It focuses on common-sense practices that can help you lead the healthiest, happiest life possible.

Natural Hygiene teaches you how to effectively manage all aspects of a healthful lifestyle—diet; exercise; rest and sleep; home and work environment; stress management; and psychology—and offers guidelines for *living in harmony with Nature.*

The premise of Natural Hygiene is that *health is normal*—the way we ought to be all the time. That outlook also is expressed in the phrase, *"Health through healthful living."* Natural Hygiene also recognizes that *healing is a biological process,* and that your body is capable of defending, regulating, and healing itself, if given the proper conditions.

The Natural Hygiene Diet, which has been compiled from the pages of the award-winning *Health Science* magazine, will teach you how to design a healthful diet tailored especially for you. A healthful diet can often play a major role in helping to maximize your health to the fullest extent possible. *The Natural Hygiene Diet* will motivate you to start and *maintain* a healthful diet *for life.* This book also will explain some of the tenets of the American Natural Hygiene Society—an extraordinary organization that can offer you a support system while you are making changes.

The American Natural Hygiene Society has promoted the principles and practices of Natural Hygiene for more than 50 years. One of the important aspects of the Society's work is keeping Natural Hygiene—the Science of Health—up-to-date and consistent with current scientific knowledge. *The Natural Hygiene Diet* will give you an introduction to the most up-to-date information about this enormously successful approach to eating, which dates back more than 160 years.

Offering simple, practical guidelines, *The Natural Hygiene Diet* includes information on diet and nutrition; delicious recipes; healthful weight loss; problems with most weight-loss programs; designing a diet that is right for you; eating healthfully in the "real" world; feeding healthy children; and so much more! Plus, you will find information on Natural Hygiene books, audiotapes, and videotapes; and a helpful chapter on the most commonly asked questions about Natural Hygiene.

Welcome to a new life of unprecedented health and vitality. By following the dietary and other principles of Natural Hygiene, you can begin experiencing a richer, more enjoyable, and more fulfilling life than you ever dreamed possible!

1

Who Should Read This Book?

Everyone who wants to achieve their ideal natural weight *healthfully,* and everyone who cares about their health—and the health of their loved ones—should read this book today!

Do you want to achieve your ideal weight? Do you want dynamic health for your loved ones? Are you convinced that conventional approaches to diet and weight loss don't work? If you answered "yes" to any of these questions, this book is for you!

The Natural Hygiene Diet contains an approach to diet that is not found *anywhere else.* This is not just another "diet" book—filled with quick-fix (and sometimes dangerous) gimmicks that don't work. This book is designed to teach you how to make the healthful dietary choices that will help you maximize your health potential, and change your life *forever!* It will provide you with powerful diet and nutrition information that will empower you to live a healthier, happier life than you ever thought possible.

Take charge of your diet and health!

Each year more than 800,000 people in America die from preventable diseases!

The full enjoyment of your life depends on learning how to live healthfully. It is estimated that more than 800,000 Americans die prematurely every year from diseases they could have avoided by changing their diets and lifestyles. *The Natural Hygiene Diet* will help you design a diet—tailored to meet your individual needs—that you can enjoy *for life!*

What you will learn

The Natural Hygiene Diet will teach you new and incredibly powerful concepts about diet and nutrition; the dramatic benefits of a plant-based diet; and how to

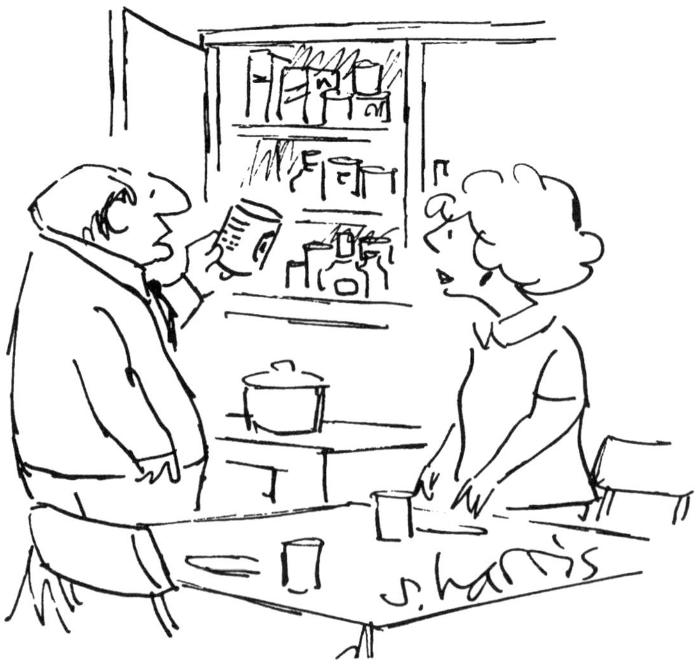

"'Clam chowder—ingredients: clams, potatoes, water, hydrolated plant protein, sodium phosphate, calcium carbonate, butylated hydroxytolune. For external use only.'"

make healthful recipes that are as delicious as they are nutritious. You also will learn how to overcome the social and psychological roadblocks to healthful eating.

The most powerful benefits you will receive may be the proven strategies that will help you succeed with your new diet, even if you have not been successful in the past. *The Natural Hygiene Diet* will show you *why* your previous "diets" did not work, and why it was not your "fault."

◆ ***Powerful strategies that work!***

The Natural Hygiene Diet will help you begin to live the life of your dreams. Say goodbye to weight problems, headaches, and digestive problems; plus, dramatically reduce your risk of the major killers in America—heart disease and cancer!

What's more, you will achieve all of this *on your own,* without dependence on any special dietary products. The most important health principle you will ever learn is that *health care is self-care!* Living and eating in a way that builds and restores health is the key. This easy-to-use book will help you reclaim the power over your own health destiny.

A totally unique approach to diet

No other diet program compares with *The Natural Hygiene Diet*. This program is unique in two ways. It is *totally* natural, and based entirely on *scientific* principles.

No need for any pills, powders, or potions!

The typical supplements, herbal extracts, energy "enhancers," internal "cleansers," appetite suppressants, high-protein diets, and other quick-fix "remedies" that dominate the "weight-loss" field are nowhere to be found in *The Natural Hygiene Diet.* Instead, you will find practical, no-nonsense advice on how to eat in a way that leads to *your* natural, ideal body weight—and helps you in your quest to maximize your health.

No need for "dieting" or deprivation

The good news about the Natural Hygiene approach is that it is not a "diet" at all, and you do not have to deprive yourself. In fact, you may even end up eating *more* than you were eating before. The big difference is that now you will be eating the foods that are designed to keep you healthfully slim.

Enjoy a wide range of food choices!

Don't be misled by those who mistakenly say that eating healthfully means a diet of limited choices and bland foods. Nothing could be farther from the truth! Healthful nutrition is not about deprivation or about eating less. It is about eating *well,* and enjoying the vibrant tastes, colors, aromas, and presentation of delicious natural foods.

Time for action

Now is the time to begin your new life. Gear up your sense of adventure, and open the door to the new diet and nutrition possibilities that will transform your enjoyment of life!

▼ ▼ ▼ ▼ ▼

In the next chapter, you will learn why the standard American diet can make you "fat for life."

2

Do You Want to Be Fat for Life?

Would you like to eat whatever you want whenever you want it? Would you like your exercise program to be as easy as pressing the remote control button on your channel-changer? If you answered "Yes!" to these questions, you need to know about an exciting new diet program called "Fat for Life!"

The *Fat for Life* program allows you to do whatever comes easiest for you—no thought or effort is required! Millions of Americans swear by the *Fat for Life* program, and it was recently announced that—for the first time in history—the majority of adults in the United States are obese. The *Fat for Life* program is really catching on.

The success of the *Fat for Life* program is not surprising when you consider that—in spite of the fact that at least 75-80% of all deaths in the United States are attributable to unhealthful diet and lifestyle choices—government officials, doctors, and even health associations often insist that the standard American diet is "healthy!"

Three out of four deaths are attributable to unhealthy diet and lifestyle!

But, if the *Fat for Life* program is so "healthy," why is it that if you are on it, all you reasonably can hope for is that you will be among the lucky one-in-five Americans who won't suffer unnecessary illness and premature death—from cancer, heart disease, stroke, diabetes, arthritis, and osteoporosis? The sad truth is that most people—even most physicians—are really in the dark when it comes to diet and nutrition.

Fortunately, you do not have to end up *Fat for Life*. There is an easy-to-understand approach to weight loss, and it doesn't involve any pills, powders, potions, or other gimmicks. It involves learning how to eat and to exercise in ways that are consistent with our natural history. That means eating a diet consisting of whole natural foods. It also means engaging in frequent, moderate exercise.

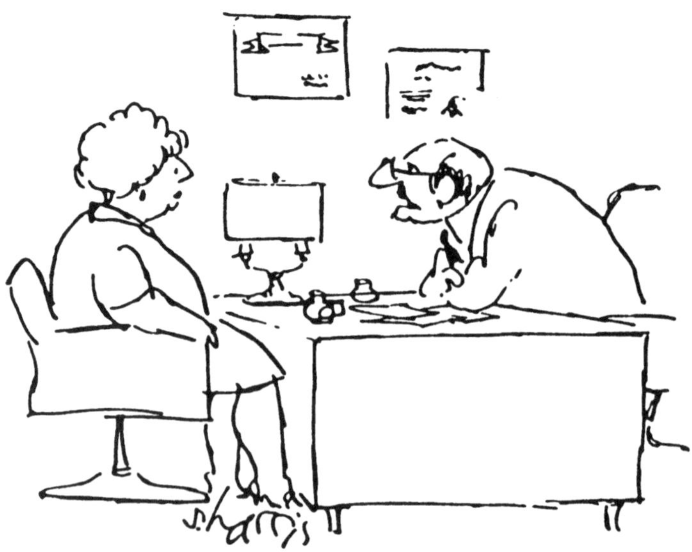

"It's partly glandular...and partly 8,500 calories per day."

Why most diets don't work

One reason that "diets" don't work is that they contain foods that were never present in the natural environment! As a result, these foods—such as bread, cheese, crackers, "low-fat" chocolate shakes, margarine, and "light" beer—have the ability to fool the brain's natural appetite mechanisms. When this happens, people tend to over-consume, and that over-consumption is stored as fat. It is just about as simple as that.

Our brains are built to sense the caloric value of foods we eat. When we have eaten enough, our hunger drive is designed to shut down naturally. Notice that you have never "accidentally" eaten fifty apples. Your body "keeps count," and shuts your hunger down at about the appropriate moment. The brain mechanism that organizes this feat is called the satiety mechanism. It was built into our psychology over countless generations, as part of our natural, biological heritage. All creatures need to know both when they are "hungry" and when they are "full," so that they can behave most effectively. ← ***Key idea!***

The satiety mechanism appears to depend upon two types of receptors in the mouth and stomach. These are *stretch receptors,* which give your brain information about how "stretched out" your stomach is, and *nutrient receptors,* which tell you the caloric density of the food you have eaten. Notice that if you eat four pounds of raw salad, you may feel "full" in terms of being "stretched out," but the nutrient receptors in your stomach also will be saying, "Hey, that was 'OK,' but it wasn't nearly enough! Get me some calories, or I'm going to continue to complain!" You might feel "stretched out," but still hungry.

Two important mechanisms tell us when to stop eating!

To be satiated, or hunger-satisfied, we have to have our stomachs both stretched out and filled with some "real" calories. In our ancestors' environment, the foods had moderate caloric density—that is, those foods both stretched the stomach *and* caused significant nutrient signaling to the brain. People couldn't easily overeat on foods of moderate density because the stretching of their stomachs would hurt. Our ancestors ate everything they could, until they felt full, and then stopped eating! They never worried about overeating and getting fat (which might have been dangerous in a natural setting). They didn't need to be concerned about this—because on a natural diet, people rarely get fat.

Processed foods

Key idea! ➡ Modern, processed foods tend to be more calorically dense than natural foods, and this can fool our satiety mechanism! When people eat substantial quantities of

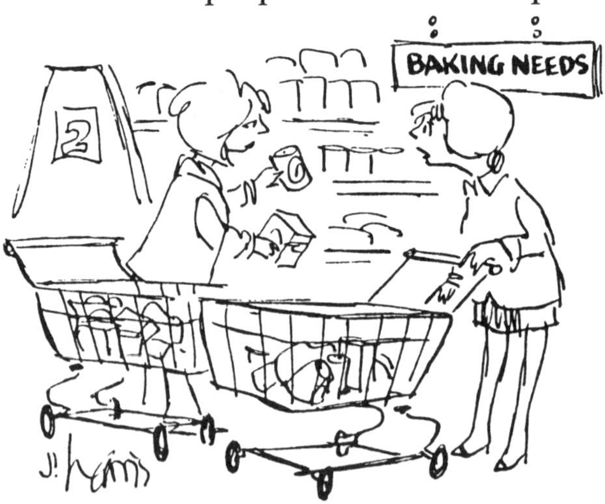

"$2.49 a pound for dilauril thiodipropionate? I think I'll switch to potassium metabisulfate."

processed foods, it is quite natural for them to overeat because the stretch receptors in their stomachs are not getting much chance to signal "enough"—until too much has been eaten.

Let's look at the caloric density of some popular foods. Raw vegetables, such as salads, contain about 100 calories per pound. Cooked vegetables, such as carrots, contain about 200 calories per pound. Fresh fruits contain about 300 calories per pound, and starchy vegetables and grains contain about 500 calories per pound. But breads, pizza, ice cream, and other processed products are usually between 1000-1500 calories per pound!

◆ ***Processed foods are packed with calories!***

Easy to overeat

A pound of bread, for example, has about 1200 calories! Because of processing, bread is a more concentrated product than grains or starchy vegetables. Therefore, when eating bread, there will be less stretch receptor activity in the stomach to signal "satiety" than if you were eating the original grains, given the same caloric intake!

Some examples might make this easier to understand. Which is easier to eat: a pint of ice cream, or five pounds of cooked carrots? Which is more likely to make you feel full: a pound of pizza, or eight pounds of cooked broccoli? Four ounces of chocolate, or three large baked potatoes? You can see that overeating is easy to do if concentrated, processed foods are prominent in the diet. Meats are also very concentrated—one of the few naturally concentrated sources of calories that some people eat. Meat consumption was probably relatively unusual in the natural environment, and it packed a big punch at about 1200 calories per pound.

In today's world, the *Fat for Life* crowd is eating a diet that predominately consists of processed foods and meat, fish, fowl, eggs, and dairy products. This guarantees that the caloric density of the average American's diet is much, much greater than his or her appetite machinery is "built" to handle! Any creature given a diet that is more concentrated than is appropriate for its design will tend to overeat, and get fat. Birds eating processed foods, for example, may fatten up to the point that they can no longer fly.

Given this perspective, it is hardly a surprise that over 50% of U.S. adults are obese, and another significant percentage are well above their optimum weight.

Remarkable new approach to weight loss

Natural foods are best for weight loss! ➨

A key strategy in any successful weight-loss program is to operate your body in the way it was meant to be operated. A top priority of this strategy is to eat a diet consisting of whole natural foods—fresh fruits and vegetables, with the variable addition of whole grains, raw nuts and seeds, and legumes. In addition to the many other health benefits, this dietary strategy will cause sufficient stretch receptor activity, resulting in satiety. With this dietary strategy, significant overeating is much less likely to occur.

At lunch and dinner, it is best if you eat your meals in a particular order. First, eat a large, raw vegetable salad. Steamed vegetables should be eaten next. Finally, eat starchy vegetables and whole grains. There is a reason for this recommendation. Once a person gets a taste of higher-calorie foods (such as cooked grains), lower-calorie foods (such as raw salad) are suddenly less appealing. This can result in less salad and vegetable consumption, which, in turn, can cause an overall increase of the meal's caloric density. By starting with the least caloric foods first—when you are the most hungry—more low-density food will be consumed. This will result in more stretching of the stomach, which will help you feel "full," making you less likely to overeat.

Using this strategy, there is little need to be concerned about portion size. There is truly no need to "go hungry." By consuming the majority of calories from moderately-concentrated, unprocessed, whole, natural foods, most of the "fat battle" is easily won. Combined with a moderate exercise program, this strategy really works—just as Nature intended.

The Center for Conservative Therapy in Penngrove, Calif. reports that "overweight patients tend to lose about

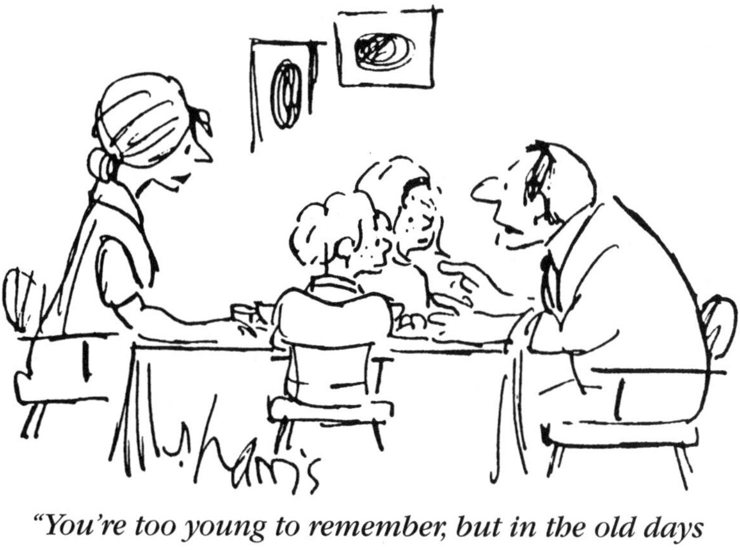

"You're too young to remember, but in the old days you could tell the vegetables apart by taste."

two pounds per week using this strategy." While most medical researchers would consider that level of weight loss to be "miraculous," Dr. Alan Goldhamer, the Center's Director, takes it all in stride. "We don't consider it 'miraculous' at all," he says. "We simply are very pleased to see our patients consistently rewarded for following our 'uncommon sense' approach to weight loss."

Exercise is not the key issue for weight loss! ➡

Some people place a tremendous emphasis on exercise for weight loss. Exercise is a useful and important adjunct to healthful living and to weight control, but exercise alone is not enough. In fact, many people who exercise almost constantly still can fail to lose weight.

At the Center for Conservative Therapy, they recommend that patients engage in moderate exercise four to five times per week and encourage patients to exercise moderately almost every day, if they have the time. "Moderate exercise," according to Dr. Goldhamer, "means an

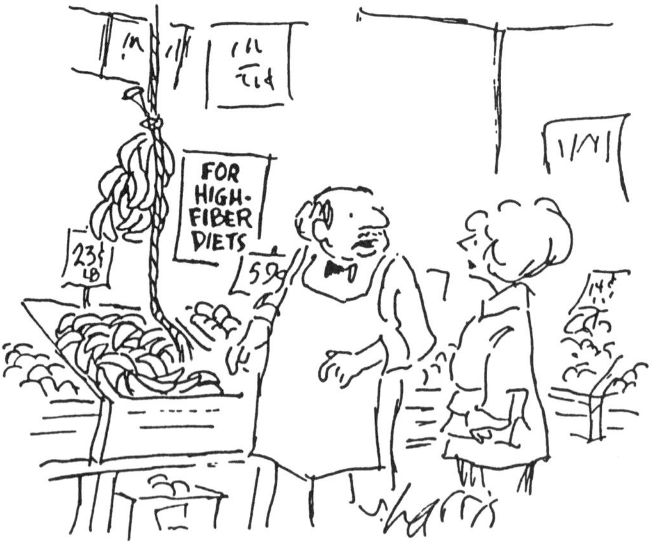

"Not the bananas—the rope."

activity that causes you to have to work at it a bit. If you are an Olympic marathoner, it might mean a five-mile run. For most of our overweight patients, however, it probably means a brisk twenty to thirty minute walk."

The success of this approach may seem "too good to be true." That is because, while the diet and exercise strategies are very simple and easy to understand, they sometimes are difficult to implement. Many factors can get in the way, but the most potent obstacle that you face in conquering the *Fat for Life* challenge is your built-in "energy conservation programming."

Programmed for convenience foods

All animals, including humans, have energy conservation programming built into their nervous systems. The nature of this programming differs from species to species, but it is always there, nonetheless.

Migratory birds, for example, will fly in a characteristic "V" pattern, so that they can use each other's bodies to break the wind, and save calories. Many fish swim in schools, saving calories riding in each other's wake. And predators all over the world are found to pick on the "weak," enabling them to get the greatest number of calories for the least amount of effort expended.

Programmed to eat high-calorie foods!

Humans, too, have this type of programming as part of human nature. We are programmed to want to get as many calories as we can, with the least possible effort! This is great programming for humans living in an environment of scarcity, which is where almost all humans lived until just the last few decades. Now, however, most of us living in the modern Western world are no longer living in an environment of scarcity. However, our natural programming is still with us—encouraging us to eat as much as we can with as little effort as possible! Is it any wonder that obesity is an epidemic within industrialized societies?

Key idea! ➡ Your "natural" tendencies may be to eat the most concentrated foods available—and to exercise as little as possible. But you needn't be a slave to these tendencies. People often are able to "over-ride" them with some moderate effort. You can "use your head" to think ahead when it comes to your health and fitness. Plan ahead to have plenty of whole natural foods conveniently available at all times, and schedule time to engage in regular, moderate exercise.

No need for miracles

You do not need a "miracle" to have a healthy, trim body. But you need to understand and respect how you were naturally designed to live. You were designed to consume a diet of whole natural foods—and to engage in moderate, regular exercise. Your energy conservation programming may make it seem "unnatural" to live this way, but that is only because of the modern environment. Progress has made unhealthful living all too easy. You do not need to follow the herd, which is headed toward fatness and failure. By implementing these simple strategies, you can join the fortunate few who are fit—not fat—for life!

▼ ▼ ▼ ▼ ▼

In the next chapter, you will learn about the dangers and drawbacks of many popular diets.

3

Is Your Diet Killing You?

In spite of the hundreds of millions of dollars spent on diets and "reducing" programs, plus the millions more spent on health clubs and exercise equipment, the United States has the most obese population in history.

What's worse, rather than taking an honest look at what causes obesity, Americans are still looking for a magic diet or some other gimmick.

Unfortunately, diets don't work because no matter how much weight you lose while you are *on* a diet, it comes right back when you go *off*. And some diets can be very dangerous to your health.

If you are serious about losing weight, you must make *permanent* lifestyle and diet changes that you are willing to live with for the rest of your life. The good news is that as soon as you develop the right eating and exercise habits, a slim, healthy body will be yours *automatically*—and *naturally*. ← ***Key idea!***

You probably already know from experience that the conventional "solution" to being overweight—low-calorie dieting—just doesn't work. But you may not know why. For the vast majority of people, being overweight is not caused by *how much* they eat, but by *what* they eat.

Researchers have found that overweight people eat about the same amount of *calories* as thin people. What makes overweight people overweight is not that they eat so much more, but that they get *a much higher percentage of their calories from fat and refined carbohydrates.* As long as you are eating fatty foods and refined carbohydrates, you won't be able to lose weight.

Our natural sweet tooth

Fresh fruit is essential for good health!

We are designed by Nature to see, grasp, eat, and enjoy the flavor of colorful, *sweet* fruits. Fruit is an essential part of our diets, absolutely necessary for us to maintain health.

Our natural desire to consume sweets was not intended to lead us to candy bars and ice cream. We need to satisfy our sweet tooth with fresh, natural fruits and other plant substances that supply us not only with carbohydrates, but with the *full complement* of nutrients we need.

"Foodless" foods

Processed carbohydrates (such as bread and cake) are just not the same as fruit. Unlike natural fruits, which have a full complement of nutrients, processed carbohydrates lack fiber, phytonutrients, vitamins, and minerals, which have been lost in processing. Eating these fragmented and unbalanced foods causes many problems—especially for those trying to lose weight. Because processed carbohydrates are lacking in fiber, they are absorbed too rapidly, causing wide swings in glucose. Also, because of the missing fiber, these foods don't make you feel "full," so you tend to want to eat more. And, because so much of the vitamin and mineral content of these foods has been lost during processing, naturally you crave more food to make up for the missing nutrients.

In contrast, when you eat mostly natural plant foods (such as fruits, vegetables, and beans), you avoid these problems. These plant foods are rich in both carbohydrates and water-soluble fibers. The fibers slow down glucose absorption and control the rate of digestion. Because of the natural fibers, and because precious vitamins, minerals, and other food factors haven't been lost through processing, natural plant foods will fill you faster—and you

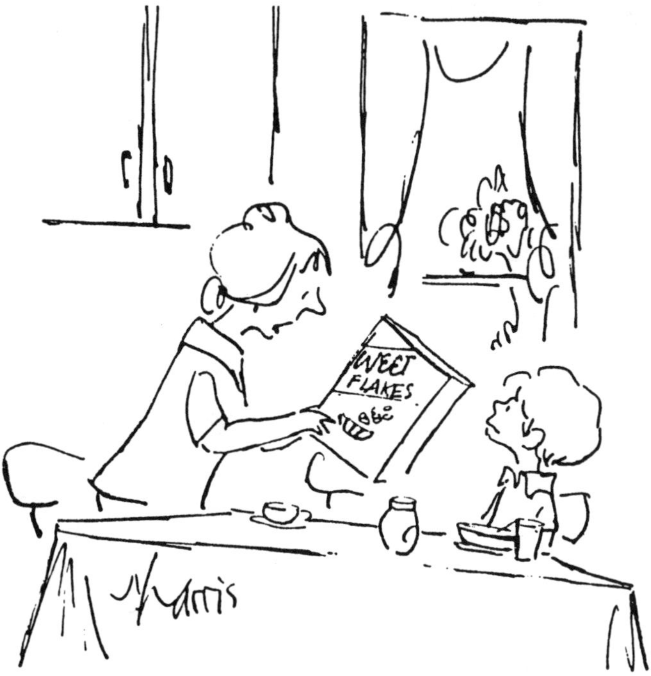

"It looks like truth in packaging has begun: One four-ounce serving provides four ounces of empty calories."

won't suffer from cravings soon after. Natural plant foods are usually carbohydrate-rich, but they also contain protein and fats. For example, vegetables contain an average of 25% of calories from protein. Eating food as it was designed by Nature is the easiest way to maintain your optimum healthy weight.

Confusion about nutrition

With all of the scientific data available today, including massive investigational studies on human health and diet, you would think that people would know what food is best to eat, and why. But people are still very confused about diet and nutrition.

Part of the problem is that most of us are slow to make changes, especially when it involves our person-

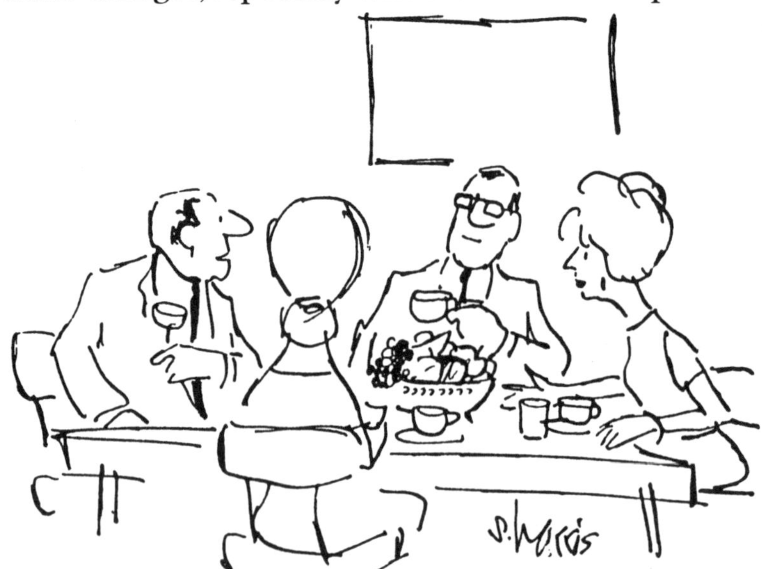

"No more, thanks. I've had my minimum daily requirement of DDT."

al habits and family traditions. The eating habits of most Americans, while seemingly an outgrowth of family traditions, have been subtly and not-so-subtly influenced by commercial interests in collusion with the government.

The egg producers, the sugar industry, the meat industry, and the dairy industry all have used heavy political and lobbying activities to influence the way government—on the local, state, and federal levels—deals with food issues. This dangerous marriage of corporate self-interest and government policy may result in the deaths of 300,000 or more Americans each year.

Politics and economics, rather than science, dictate public policy on diet and nutrition. Prevailed upon by lobbyists wielding tremendous economic power, the government continues to make dietary recommendations that have been at odds with nutritional science for decades. The food industry does not want change in the nation's eating habits. After all, its major players have spent fifty years and countless billions of dollars training us not only to eat their products, but to think they are *necessary* for health. The tragedy is that the opposite is true. Not only are these foods *not* necessary, it is almost *impossible* to eat these products and stay healthy.

"Four food groups" myths

Fifty years ago, the U.S. Department of Agriculture (USDA) began promoting the so-called "four basic food groups," with meat and dairy products in the number one and two spots on the list. This program, which more accurately could have been called "the four food myths," was taught in every classroom in America, with posters advocating a diet loaded with animal protein, fat, and cholesterol. This government propaganda, which most of us learned as children, was based on the economic interests of powerful food manufacturers.

The results of this program were dramatic—in more ways than one. Americans began eating more and more animal foods. Unfortunately, the "four basic food groups" campaign has coincided with the fastest growing cancer epidemic in history, and heart attack rates have soared.

Kicking a lifelong habit

Corporate menu planning and your health!

Since early childhood, we have been indoctrinated with incorrect nutritional and dietary advice—and the scandal continues. Even after decades of scientific research refuting the USDA guidelines, the latest USDA recommendations—the "food pyramid"—are only a slight improvement. They still reinforce the dietary errors that people have become accustomed to making.

Key idea! ➨

In light of all the scientific data available, the USDA's recommendations are a disgrace. Many large-scale epidemiological studies have shown conclusively that certain plant foods can play a major role in protecting the body against the diseases that kill at least 300,000 Americans each year. There is no longer any question about the importance of fruits and vegetables in the diet. The greater the quantity and assortment of fruits and vegetables consumed, the lesser the incidence of heart attacks and cancer.

Heart disease and many cancers, which very accurately could be called "diseases of nutritional ignorance," kill more than 85% of all Americans. If we were not so misinformed, and were armed with accurate information about diet and nutrition, we could realistically

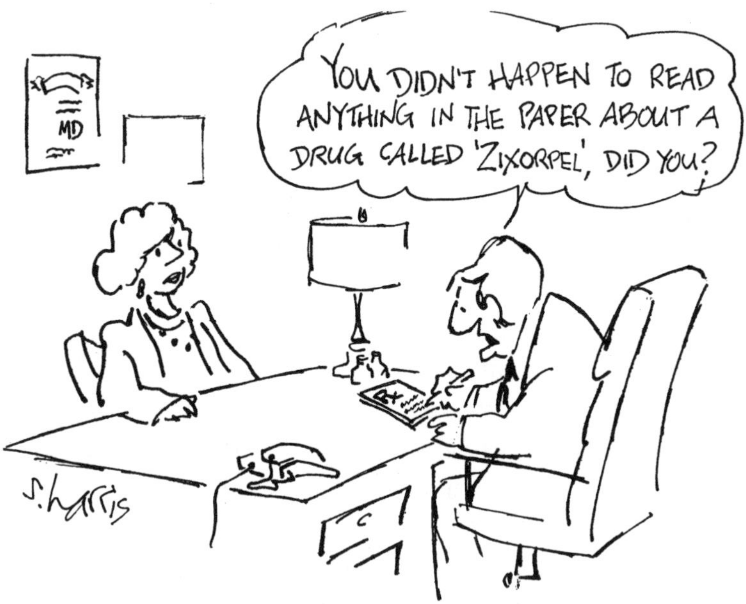
YOU DIDN'T HAPPEN TO READ ANYTHING IN THE PAPER ABOUT A DRUG CALLED 'ZIXORPEL', DID YOU?
MD
S. harris

expect to add ten to twenty-five *quality* years to our lives. And, at the same time, we would not ever have to worry about becoming overweight again. When you eat the right foods and engage in a moderate exercise program, being overweight is almost impossible.

On the conventional diet most Americans eat, with most of the calories coming from refined carbohydrates and animal foods, it is just about as easy to get sick as to get fat. At present, Americans consume about 50% of calories from fiberless animal foods and another 40% of calories from refined carbohydrates. Americans only consume 5-8% of calories from fruits and vegetables. So it should not come as any surprise that we have such a sick society—with medical costs out of control—and an epidemic of the diseases related to nutritional illiteracy, especially heart attacks and cancer.

High-protein diets

More than 50% of all Americans are overweight, so it is not surprising that diet and weight-loss books abound. Each promises advice on how to become a new, *thinner,* you.

The success of these books can be measured by their popularity (the number of books sold) or by how well the diet programs work (how many pounds you reasonably can expect to lose on the diet). But there are many more important considerations than these.

Key idea! ➡ Weight loss and overall health are inseparable. A weight-loss program can be considered successful only if the weight loss is permanent, if it is safe, and if it promotes overall health. Temporary weight loss is of little or no benefit, especially if it compromises your health.

Unfortunately, many of the best-selling weight-loss programs have serious drawbacks. But their popularity is evidence that people are looking for a quick, effortless way to lose weight without having to curtail their dangerous love affair with rich, unhealthful foods.

Problems with high-protein diets are serious!

Two of these books, *Dr. Atkins' New Diet Revolution,* by Robert Atkins, M.D., and *The Zone,* by Barry Sears, Ph.D., advocate high-protein weight-loss plans that include diets with significantly more animal protein than already is being consumed by the average American. Americans eat almost 50% of their calories from animal products. This nutritional extravagance has resulted in a tragic skyrocketing of cancer and heart disease rates during the last 50 years.

Dr. Atkins recommends that you eat an abundance of high-protein foods and eliminate carbohydrates from your diet. The goal is rapid weight loss, and the program is "successful" because you can lose weight quickly. But can we call a diet "successful" if a key component of it—high consumption of animal products—brings with it such serious health risks?

Hundreds of scientific studies have documented the link between animal protein and various cancers. The evidence of this link is now as solid as the link between smoking and lung cancer. While it would be wrong to say that animal foods are the sole cause of cancer, it is now clear that the most powerful effect on cancer risk is increased consumption of animal products and decreased consumption of fresh produce.

A meat-based, low-fiber diet that includes no fruit or starchy vegetables will almost *double your risk* of certain cancers, especially meat-sensitive cancers, such as colon cancer. Stomach and esophageal cancer, for example, are linked to populations that do not consume sufficient fruit.

◆ ***A diet to die for!***

Excess weight a real problem

An argument can be made for the usefulness of diets such as the one advocated by Atkins because they do result in weight loss. Being overweight is such a health risk that there are some real health benefits one receives from losing weight, even if the mode of weight loss places the person at increased risk. Losing weight—even on a high-protein, high-fat, low-fiber diet—will lower triglycerides, decrease insulin resistance, and lower blood pressure.

These high-protein diets forbid the eating of refined carbohydrates, junk food, and the nutritionally depleted white pasta and white bread that most Americans consume in large quantities. They also recommend that the dieter consume hundreds of dollars worth of nutritional supplements each month. The conventional American diet is so unhealthful and fattening that diets like these may offer more micronutrient density than the diet the person was on previously.

The menu plans advocated by Sears are an improvement over Atkins' because they permit small amounts of fruit and starchy vegetables. The goal of this book is to teach people how to keep their hormone levels in the right "zone" by eating equal amounts of fats, carbohydrates, and proteins at each meal. Some people can benefit from this, but there are so many other factors to consider.

Key idea! ➨ Sears evidently fails to realize that animal proteins and plant proteins are vastly different macronutrients with a huge difference in biochemical effects. He ignores the wealth of information showing that it is plant proteins, not animal proteins, that lower cholesterol and reduce cancer risk.

Benefits of plant foods

Phytochemicals and plant fibers are a hot area of interest in nutritional research today. Phytochemicals, often called chemopreventive compounds, now number in the thousands and have been shown to have the powerful effects of improving human immune function and preventing cancer.

Plant fibers—the undigestible and unabsorbed part of the plant foods—are now looked at in a completely different way than in the past. It is now understood that it is not merely the *amount* of fiber in the diet that protects against cancer; the primary importance is the *vari-*

ety of fiber consumed. Our digestive tract is teeming with bacteria that convert these fibers into numerous essential fatty acids and other nutrients. These food factors are essential for optimal health and protection against various cancers, especially colon cancer. In other words, you can not just add psyllium powder to an American diet and think your fiber needs will be met; you must eat a variety of soluble and insoluble plant fibers from an assortment of natural foods.

Sears seems so oblivious to the powerful, protective, anti-cancer effects of phytonutrients and various plant fibers that he equates a healthful, vegetarian diet with a candy bar. He comes to this astonishing conclusion based on a superficial similarity in the ratio of protein to carbohydrates in each.

Sears is on the mark when he identifies pasta and bread as poor foods. He correctly points out that just because a diet is low in fat and nearly free of animal foods does not

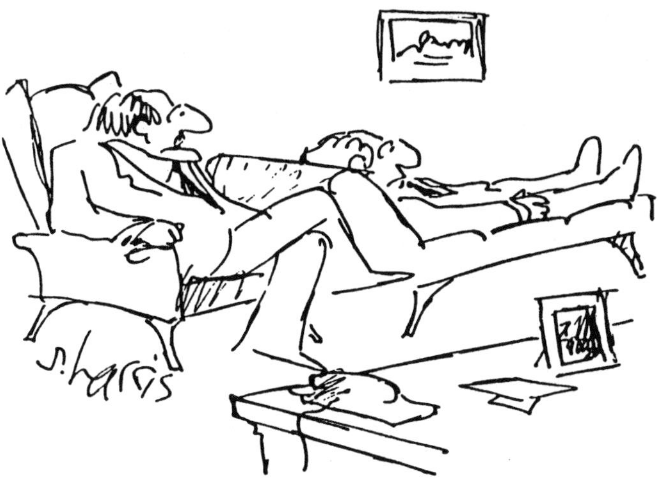

"Forget Freud. Thoreau is the answer. Work in your garden. Eat beans and squash. Write about it."

mean it is a healthful one. For a diet to be truly healthful, it must be low in fat, low in animal protein, and rich in nutrient-dense foods.

Sears' diet plan is an improvement over the diet most Americans consume because it removes the base of the USDA pyramid—refined grains—and, therefore, encourages more fruit and vegetable consumption. He discourages eating the fattier, more dangerous animal foods, such as red meat, egg yolks, and fatty cheeses, and he discourages eating junk food.

But Sears' diet is far from the best. Any person with a daily consumption of twelve ounces of animal products is asking for trouble. There is a linear relationship between animal food consumption and both heart disease and cancer. Sears' goal of about 100 grams of animal protein a day places his devotees at the highest

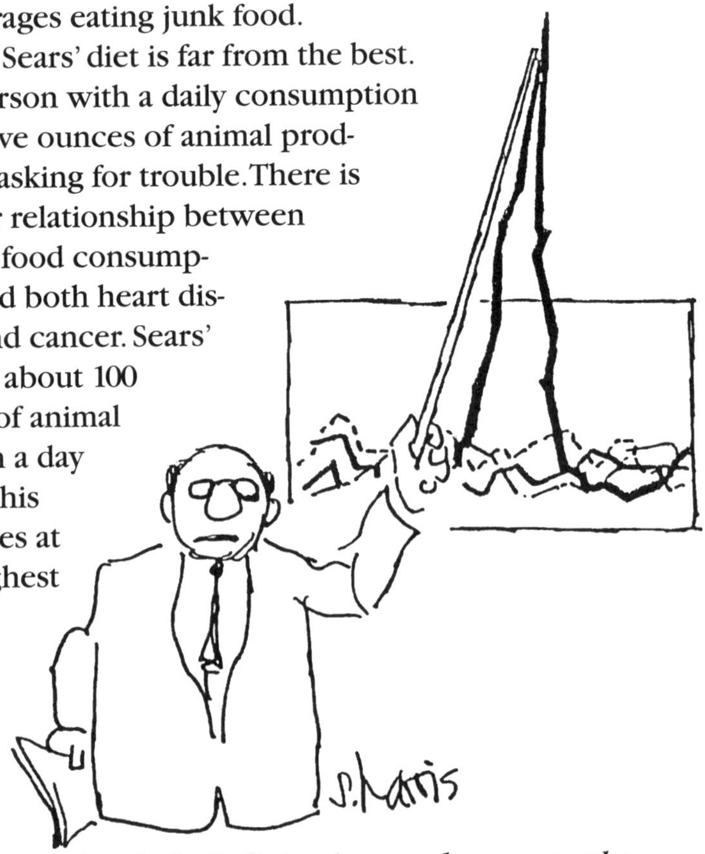

"Whereas the alcoholic living in an urban area, who eats high cholesterol foods and smokes 3 packs a day..."

worldwide consumption of animal protein. Accordingly, they should expect to experience similar incidences of the killer diseases that afflict Americans.

Sears actually argues in favor of a primitive, natural food based diet. But he misses the boat when he replaces the empty-calories of the refined carbohydrates that most Americans consume with animal foods, rather than with fruit, vegetables, beans, nuts, and seeds. Inexplicably, Sears never counts vegetables as a significant source of protein, and he classifies greens (such as kale, broccoli, Swiss chard, and turnip greens), beans, and lentils as carbohydrates, even though most of their calories come from protein.

It is disheartening that so many people will attempt to lose weight on programs that contradict everything we know about cancer prevention and longevity. High-fat, high-animal protein diets have almost no fiber, they utilize the precise foods (animal products) known to be the primary causes of cancer and heart attacks, and they specifically exclude the foods that have been shown to prevent cancer—such as fruit, yellow and orange vegetables, and beans.

The ideal diet

The research is clear. The *ideal* diet for health and weight loss must significantly *reduce or eliminate* animal products and significantly *increase* fruit and raw vegetables as well. The most consistent finding in the nutritional literature throughout every epidemiological study is that as fruit and vegetable consumption increases in the diet, chronic diseases and premature deaths decrease. ← ***Key idea!***

The reason that populations on very low-fat diets (such as those studied in the massive China-Oxford-Cornell

Study) have such low rates of cancer and heart disease is not merely because the diets are low in fat, but because the vast majority of the foods people are consuming are unrefined plant foods.

The way to lose weight effortlessly, improve your quality of life, enhance longevity, and decrease the risks of heart attack and cancer is to learn to avoid refined carbohydrates and significantly reduce or eliminate animal foods. By taking these steps, you will lose weight, significantly increase your health level, and prolong your life.

▼ ▼ ▼ ▼ ▼

In the next chapter, you will learn the powerful, yet easy to understand, basics of the Natural Hygiene diet!

4

The Natural Hygiene Diet

The American Natural Hygiene Society recommends a whole-food, plant-based diet (organically grown, whenever possible) that consists primarily of fresh, uncooked fruits and vegetables; steamed vegetables; baked potatoes, yams, and hard squashes; and the variable addition of (raw, unsalted) nuts, whole grains, and legumes, designed to meet individual needs. It recommends the avoidance of all animal products—meat, fish, fowl, eggs, and dairy products—as well as added oil, salt, sugar, and most other highly-processed foods.

The Natural Hygiene diet is unique in that it advocates that the greatest portion of the diet (by volume) be fresh, uncooked fruits and vegetables. Other vegetarian and vegan (total vegetarian) diets typically make cooked grains their focus.

← Important concept!

The Natural Hygiene diet has been helping people for more than 160 years, but only during the past twenty years has its effectiveness been confirmed. An overwhelming number of scientific studies now support the extraordinary benefits of a plant-based diet. Scientists continue to thoroughly document the link between the consumption of animal products and heart disease, cancer, diabetes, osteoporosis, kidney disease, and other serious problems.

The American Natural Hygiene Society has been promoting a vegetarian diet longer (since 1948) than any other health organization in the United States. By contrast, the medical establishment has only recently, and reluctantly, begun to acknowledge the inseparable relationship between diet and health.

Dietary excess is a significant factor in many diseases.

Furthermore, contrary to what the food supplement industry would like you to think, diseases from nutritional deficiency are not nearly as common as degenerative diseases from dietary *excess*—especially of animal products and highly-processed, "foodless" foods.

The major deficiency most Americans should be concerned about is the lack of fiber in their diets because they don't eat enough fruits, vegetables, whole grains, and legumes. Meat and dairy products do not contain any fiber, and foods made from refined grains—such as white bread, white rice, and white pasta—have had their fiber removed. Fiber deficiency leads to many common health problems, such as constipation, hemorrhoids, varicose veins, hiatus hernia, and hypoglycemia. Lack of fiber in the diet makes diabetes much harder to control, and is a major factor in increasing the incidence of cancer, especially colon and breast cancer.

Science supports vegetarian diet

The scientific literature clearly confirms that a diet derived exclusively from whole, natural foods provides you with both the quantity and quality of nutrients you need for optimum health, so long as you eat enough to meet your individual caloric needs. So, if you like to eat, you'll love the Natural Hygiene diet!

The nutrients you need include: *protein* (for its essential amino acid components); *fat* (for its essential fatty acid components); *complex carbohydrates* (as a clean-burning source of fuel); *vitamins* (for their role as catalysts and cofactors); *minerals* (that serve as structural components); *fiber* (as a necessary source of roughage); *water* (the universal solvent); and *phytochemicals* (for the possible role they play in supporting and protecting the body).

On the specific issue of protein—a healthful, calorie-sufficient, whole-food, plant-based diet will supply ample amounts of high-quality protein per day.

Problems with eating animal products

Human beings are not designed for a diet based on meat!

Unlike other animals that include meat in their diets, humans are unable to break down uric acid. This is due to the fact that we do not possess the necessary enzyme, uricase. This inability to break down uric acid leads to an increased possibility of its accumulating in the body when animal products are eaten. Uric acid is an intermediary product of metabolism that is associated with various pathological states, including gout.

The human liver, unlike the livers of carnivores, can process only a limited amount of cholesterol. If significant amounts of animal products are consumed, cholesterol levels rise, along with an increased risk of developing atherosclerosis. Clearly, the human liver was not designed to handle the large amounts of animal prod-

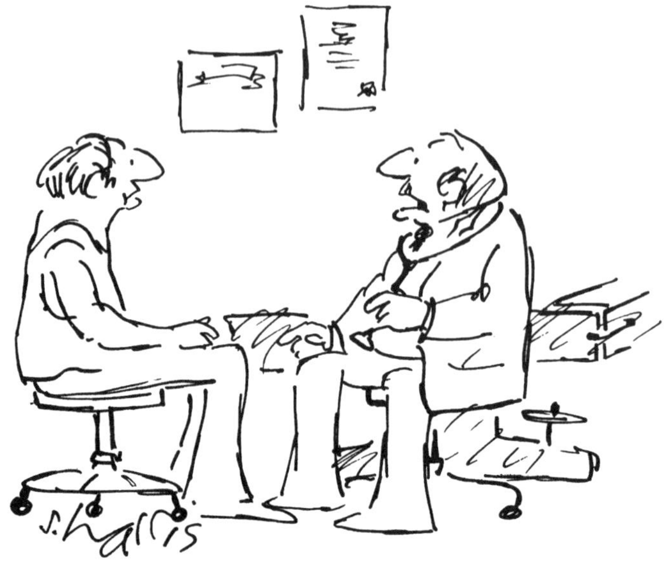

"Amazing—you have the heart of a 375-year-old man."

ucts that are consumed by most Americans.

Uncooked or improperly cooked meat, fish, fowl, and dairy products are the sources of parasites and contamination—such as trichinosis (found in pork and pork-contaminated beef) and salmonellosis (found in chicken, milk products, and other contaminated animal products).

The price we pay for meat

Vegetarians use fewer healthcare services and spend less time in hospitals than people who eat meat.

Most of us know how much a fast-food hamburger costs, but few of us realize how much meat eating costs Americans in annual healthcare expenditures.

According to a report published in the November, 1995 issue of *Preventive Medicine,* meat eating results in as much as $61 *billion* in annual healthcare costs due to increases in heart disease, hypertension, cancer, diabetes, gallstones, obesity-related problems, and food-borne illness.

Meat eaters also are more likely to smoke and drink alcohol, further jeopardizing their health. The medical costs attributable to smoking are generally considered to be $50 billion annually.

Vegetarian diet now on Uncle Sam's menu

The scientific support for vegetarianism is now so strong that even the government of the United States has had to recognize the nutritional adequacy of both the vegetarian and vegan diets. This came in the wake of the nearly fifty years of pressure from the American Natural Hygiene Society and other health groups.

United States government recognizes vegetarian and vegan diets!

Now, the government publication *Dietary Guidelines for Americans*—the nation's blueprint for nutrition programs, which is updated every five years—gives its stamp of approval to the vegetarian and vegan diets. It also states that a healthful diet can help reduce the risks of developing diseases such as heart disease, certain cancers, diabetes, stroke, and osteoporosis, as well as reduce major risk factors, such as obesity, high blood pressure, and high cholesterol.

More progress still needed

While the U.S. government has made progress in its *Dietary Guidelines for Americans,* its recommendations still show the influence of industry groups that want their products included in this influential publication. As a result, parts of the *Dietary Guidelines*

◂ Dietary guidelines in debate!

look as much like a fast-food menu as they do a scientific document.

The government's *Food Guide Pyramid,* which is included in the *Dietary Guidelines,* still recommends two-to-three servings of meat and two-to-three servings of dairy products every day, in spite of the fact that research shows that avoiding such products is safer than consuming them.

Experts ask government to end dietary focus on animal products!

Under the auspices of the Washington-based Physicians Committee for Responsible Medicine, a distinguished group of scientists and physicians has called for the government's meat- and dairy-based diet to be traded for a plant-based diet.

These physicians included the late Dr. Benjamin Spock, author of *Baby and Child Care,* which has long been the leading guide for parents; Dr. Henry Heimlich, inventor of the Heimlich maneuver and many other medical innovations; Dr. William Castelli, Director of the Framingham Heart Study; Dr. William Roberts, Editor of the *American Journal of Cardiology;* Dr. Dean Ornish, from the University of California at San Francisco; Dr. Peter Wood, of the Stanford Center for Research in Disease Prevention; Dr. Caldwell Esselstyn, Jr., of the Cleveland Clinic's Department of General Surgery; Dr. Frank Oski, Chairman of the Department of Pediatrics at Johns Hopkins University; Dr. Lawrence Kushi, of the University of Minnesota; Dr. Oliver Alabaster, Director of the Institute for Disease Prevention of the George Washington University Medical Center; Dr. Neal D. Barnard, President of the Physicians Committee for Responsible Medicine; and many others, including members of the International Association of Hygienic Physicians.

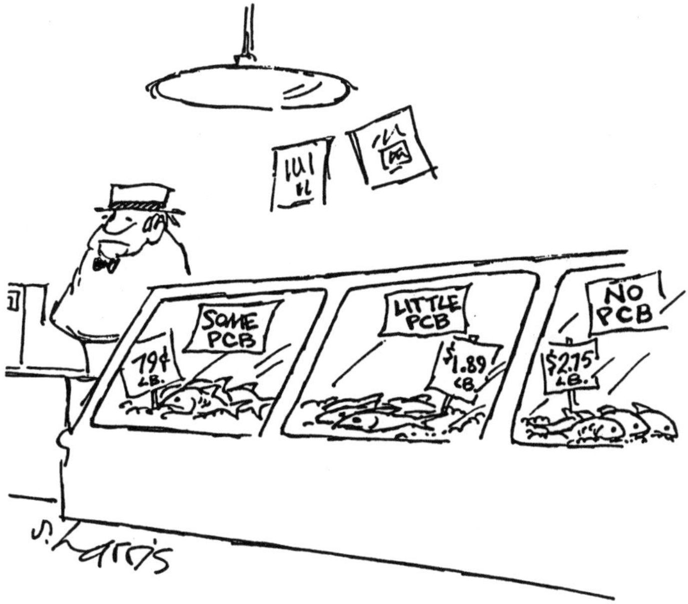

Natural Hygiene dietary recommendations

The Natural Hygiene diet is as easy to understand and to adopt as it is beautiful to see and delicious to eat. As mentioned at the beginning of this chapter, the American Natural Hygiene Society recommends a plant-based diet derived exclusively from whole natural foods and which excludes meat, fish, fowl, eggs, dairy products, added oil, salt, sugar, and most processed foods.

These recommendations alone would not make the Natural Hygiene diet special. Natural Hygiene stands apart from other vegetarian and vegan diets in that it recommends that you eat a very large portion of your diet uncooked, use a minimum of spices and other stimulants, and center your diet around fruits and vegetables, including complex starches, such as potatoes and yams, rather than concentrating primarily on grains.

Plant-based diet is your key to good health!

Natural Hygienists are the original "raw food" advocates, pointing to the joys of eating delicious, nutritious meals fresh from Nature's bountiful gardens and orchards. ("Food" from slaughterhouses and food-processing plants simply cannot compare!) Natural Hygienists recommend simply-prepared meals that help discourage overeating. In the 1930s, a popular practice known as "food combining" was devised to help people simplify their meals.

Uncooked fruits and vegetables are alive with exquisite flavors and aromas, and provide you with Nature's full palate of nutrients (vitamins, minerals, amino acids, phytochemicals, and enzymes), fiber, and water in abundance.

Eat *more!* A health-promoting diet is *high* in nutrients and *low* in calories!

Fresh fruits and vegetables are Nature's perfect foods, and they are low in calories. Raw salad vegetables—such as leaf lettuce, celery, carrots, tomatoes, sweet red peppers, broccoli, cauliflower, jicama, kohlrabi, snow peas, sweet cabbages, and cucumbers—contain (on average) only about 100 calories per pound. Fresh fruit—apples, pears, bananas, apricots, plums, nectarines, fresh figs, grapes, peaches, oranges, strawberries, blueberries, raspberries, persimmons, watermelon, cantaloupe, and countless other regional fruits—contains (on average) only about 300 calories per pound.

Although there are countless benefits from eating uncooked fruits and vegetables, the American Natural Hygiene Society does not advocate a *totally* raw-food diet. A diet made up solely of raw fruits and vegetables requires you to eat a very large volume of food to get sufficient calories to maintain weight and energy levels. Because most active adults need about 2,000 calories per day, you would need to eat at least twelve-to-fifteen pounds of fruits and vegetables each day. This is not practical for most people.

Fortunately, steamed vegetables contain (on average) about 300 calories per pound (and some people find them easier to eat); baked potatoes, yams, and hard squashes contain (on average) about 500 calories per pound; grains, such as brown rice, millet, and quinoa, also contain about 500 calories per pound; avocados (which are high in fat) contain about 800 calories per pound; and raw, unsalted nuts (which are *very* high in fat) contain about 2,500 calories per pound.

What should I eat?

When beginning to eat healthfully, a good starting point is to eat a large volume of fresh, raw fruits and vegetables (three to five pounds per day, yielding 600 to 1,100 calories) and to get enough cooked, starchy vegetables (such as potatoes, yams, and hard squashes), legumes (such as lentils, and other beans), and whole grains (such as brown rice, millet, and quinoa) so that you can maintain good strength and energy levels and not get too skinny.

A large portion of your diet should be uncooked fruits and vegetables!

Because some vegetable foods are naturally high in fat and protein, it makes sense to eat them sparingly. It is recommended that you are careful not to consume large quantities of avocado, nuts, or soy products on a daily basis.

The big picture

It is important to keep the big picture in mind when you start making dietary changes. People just starting out often focus much of their attention on insignificant

← Important tip!

points. Please don't become one of them!

It is all-too-common to hear people who have never previously given a moment's thought to health or nutrition become instant experts on such topics as "live foods," "depleted soils," "enzymes," "food combining," "supplements," and so on, minutes after first hearing about them.

Key idea! ➡ The most important step you can take to improve your diet is to eliminate or at least dramatically reduce your consumption of animal products—meat, fish, fowl, eggs, and dairy products. Improving the American diet—including a dramatic reduction or elimination of animal products—could save as many as 300,000 lives each year.

No other dietary change can produce such extraordinary benefits. Eliminate animal products from your diet *now.* Later on, you can argue all you want about minute, theoretical details.

One of the most important concepts that you will ever learn about diet and nutrition is that food is *fuel.* It is so very important that you eat to live and not live to eat.

▼ ▼ ▼ ▼ ▼

In the next chapter, you will learn practical tips on how to design a diet that meets ***your*** *individual needs.*

5

Designing a Healthful Diet That Is Right for You

It sometimes seems like everyone you talk to is trying to eat more healthfully. And, as the scientific evidence mounts in support of a whole-food, plant-based diet, more and more people want to adopt this health-promoting way of eating. But simply understanding the scientific support for your new diet is not always enough to ensure a successful transition.

Most people have questions about making a transition to healthful eating. Here are the six most frequently asked questions:

1. ***What foods should I eat?***
2. ***What foods should I avoid?***
3. ***Will my new diet meet all of my nutritional needs?***
4. ***Will I enjoy my new diet?***
5. ***How will I feel physically and emotionally?***
6. ***Can I do it?***

The answers to these questions are surprisingly easy to understand and put into practice. Once you learn a few simple principles, you will be on your way to a new way of eating that will bring more health and enjoyment than you ever might have imagined!

What's on the main menu?

You have an amazingly wide range of foods to choose from. There are countless varieties of fresh fruits; vegetables; potatoes and hard squashes; whole grains and legumes; and raw, unsalted nuts and seeds. Prepare yourself for a delightful taste adventure as you explore your new way of eating!

There is a wide range of fresh, tasty foods to choose from!

The list that follows is a sampling of some of the delicious whole, natural foods (organically grown, whenever possible) that will be the heart and soul of your new diet. For a complete description of these foods and their nutritional breakdowns, order a copy of *Dictionary of Natural Foods,* by Dr. William Esser, from the American Natural Hygiene Society. (See page 122.)

Fresh fruits

Apples, apricots, avocados, bananas, blackberries, blueberries, cantaloupes, fresh dates, elderberries, fresh figs, gooseberries, grapefruits, grapes, mangos, musk melons, nectarines, oranges, peaches, pears, persimmons, pineapples, plums, raspberries, strawberries, tangerines, watermelon, and countless other exotic fruits, such as breadfruits, carambolas, cherimoyas, guavas, jackfruits, papayas, sapadillas, sapotes, and soursops.

Fresh vegetables

Salad vegetables—such as broccoli, sweet cabbages, carrots, cauliflower, celery, corn, cucumbers, jicama, kohlrabi, leaf lettuce, sweet red peppers, snow peas, and tomatoes; plus others—such as artichokes, asparagus, beets, brussels sprouts, collards, eggplant, kale, mustard greens, okra, parsnips, rhubarb, rutabaga, spinach, summer squash, turnips, water chestnuts, and zucchini.

Potatoes and hard squashes

Many varieties of potatoes (including new, russet, white, purple, Yukon gold, and yellow Finn), sweet potatoes, yams, pumpkins, acorn squash, butternut squash, and hubbard squash.

Legumes

Chickpeas, cowpeas, green beans, green peas, lentils, lima beans, pigeonpeas, pinto beans, red beans, snap beans, soybeans, and white beans.

Grains

Brown rice, wild rice, millet, quinoa, oats, buckwheat (kasha).

Raw, unsalted nuts and seeds

Almonds, black walnuts, cashews, English walnuts, filberts, hickory nuts, macadamias, pecans, pignolias (pine nuts), pistachios, pumpkin seeds, sesame seeds, and sunflower seeds.

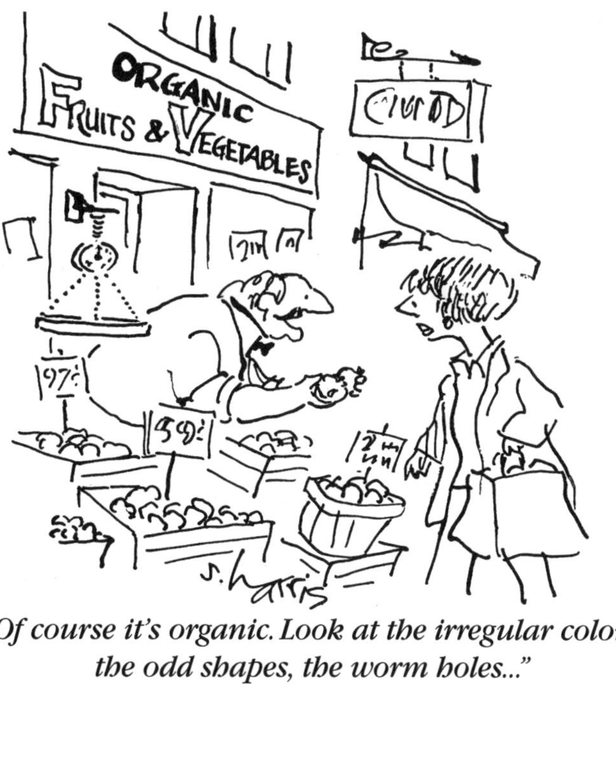

"Of course it's organic. Look at the irregular colors, the odd shapes, the worm holes..."

What foods should I avoid?

There are several categories of food you need to avoid—animal products (meat, fish, fowl, eggs, and dairy products); most processed foods; added oils, salt, and sugar; and all food additives and chemicals.

Meeting your nutritional needs

Your nutritional needs change during your lifetime!

People come in all shapes and sizes. We each have different metabolisms, different activity levels, different heights and weights, and different ages. We also have individual capacities for digestion. Because each of these factors can change during our lifetime, we need to fashion a diet that continually meets our *individual* needs.

With this in mind, two sample daily menus are described below, one for a healthy, active female, twenty-five-to-fifty years old; another for a healthy, active male, twenty-five-to-fifty years old.

Two sample one-day menus

Here is a one-day example of a health-promoting diet for a healthy, active female, twenty-five-to-fifty years old:

Breakfast:
Fresh raw fruit salad including a banana, apple, and strawberries along with celery and one ounce each of almonds and raw pumpkin seeds.

Lunch:
Large raw vegetable salad (lettuce, carrot, beets, tomato, alfalfa sprouts, peas, cucumber) with Tomato Avocado Dressing and a large plate of steamed vegetables and baked potato.

Dinner:
Raw vegetable plate (carrot, jicama, celery, cucumber) with steamed vegetables, and Brown Rice-Lentil Stew.

(For recipes, see the end of this chapter.)

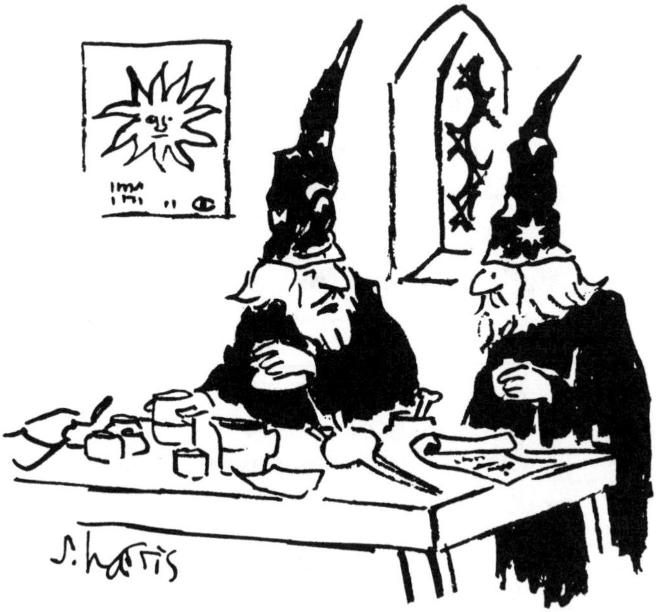

"I'm attempting to transmute calcium oxide, copper, gluconate, manganese sulfate, tyrosine, and benzaldehyde into condensed soup."

Here is a one-day example of a health-promoting diet for a healthy, active male, twenty-five-to-fifty years old:

Breakfast:
Orange juice smoothie (orange juice, banana, kiwi) and oatmeal with raisins.

Lunch:
Vegetable plate with avocado slices, steamed vegetables, and Potato-Vegetable Soup.

Dinner:
Large raw vegetable salad (lettuce, carrot, beets, tomato, alfalfa sprouts, peas, cucumber) with Tomato Avocado Dressing, a large plate of steamed vegetables, and a bowl of Split Pea–Yam Soup over brown rice.

(For recipes, see the end of this chapter.)

If additional calories are required, a fresh mixed

vegetable juice or fresh fruit could be consumed in the afternoon.

The charts on these pages show that the sample daily menus for women and men described in the text are more than adequate to meet your nutritional needs.

This chart shows that the sample daily menu on page 54 for a healthy, active female, age 25 to 50, is more than adequate!

Average daily nutrients from 1700-calorie menu

Nutrient	Amount	RDA %	Nutrient	Amount	RDA %
Calories	1695 Kc	77.0%	Vitamin C	778.5 mg	1297.0%
Protein	59.74 Gm	110.0%	Vitamin E	43.15 mg	539.0%
Histidine	1411 mg	256.0%	Vitamin K	2373 Ug	3651.0%
Isoleucine	2513 mg	386.0%	Pantothenic Acid	8.724 mg	158.0%
Methionine	759.8 mg	178.0%	Chromium	0.2111 mg	168.0%
Phenylalanine	2475 mg	521.0%	Linoleic Acid	5.553 Gm	113.0%
Threonine	2122 mg	471.0%	Magnesium	688.1 mg	245.0%
Tyrosine	1698 mg	357.0%	Potassium	7364 mg	368.0%
Leucine	3735 mg	393.0%	Copper	3.111 mg	138.0%
Lysine	3055 mg	381.0%	Iron	22.25 mg	148.0%
Tryptophan	684.2 mg	273.0%	Phosphorus	1425 mg	178.0%
Valine	2945 mg	453.0%	Manganese	9.885 mg	282.0%
Vitamin A	7447 RE	930.0%	Selenium	0.184 mg	333.0%
Thiamin B_1	1.938 mg	176.0%	Calcium	933.5 mg	116.0%
Riboflavin B_2	2.118 mg	162.0%	Cholesterol	0.0 mg	n/a
Niacin B_3	22.18 mg	147.0%	Carbohydrate	332.5 Gm	120.0%
Pyridoxine B_6	4.964 mg	310.0%	Weight	3004 Gm	n/a
Cobalamin B_{12}	0.0 Ug	0.0%	Dietary Fiber	71.46 Gm	324.0%

Percent of calories from: Protein: 13% Carbohydrate: 73% Fat: 14%

How to enjoy your new diet

How quickly you will enjoy your new diet pretty much depends on you. Some people like to jump into it all at once—and they feel great! For others, making a swift and dramatic dietary change—from a typical American diet to a Hygienic diet—might leave them feeling physically worse and emotionally deprived for a short time.

You may experience withdrawal symptoms from your old diet, and may need time to develop effective strategies to deal with friends and loved ones who feel threatened by the *new* you.

Average daily nutrients from 2500-calorie menu

Nutrient	Amount	RDA %	Nutrient	Amount	RDA %
Calories	2468 Kc	85.0%	Vitamin C	1176 mg	1960.0%
Protein	86.38 Gm	137.0%	Vitamin E	56.75 mg	567.0%
Histidine	1888 mg	272.0%	Vitamin K	2117 Ug	2646.0%
Isoleucine	3322 mg	405.0%	Pantothenic Acid	10.71 mg	194.0%
Methionine	1105 mg	206.0%	Chromium	0.169 mg	135.0%
Phenylalanine	3454 mg	576.0%	Linoleic Acid	5.625 Gm	87.0%
Threonine	2786 mg	491.0%	Magnesium	963.3 mg	275.0%
Tyrosine	2281 mg	380.0%	Potassium	9632 mg	481.0%
Leucine	5186 mg	433.0%	Copper	3.711 mg	164.0%
Lysine	3978 mg	394.0%	Iron	27.32 mg	273.0%
Tryptophan	922.4 mg	292.0%	Phosphorus	2083 mg	260.0%
Valine	3958 mg	483.0%	Manganese	14.98 mg	428.0%
Vitamin A	10144 RE	1014.0%	Selenium	0.248 mg	354.0%
Thiamin B_1	3.479 mg	231.0%	Calcium	1052 mg	131.0%
Riboflavin B_2	2.11 mg	137.0%	Cholesterol	0.0 mg	n/a
Niacin B_3	23.79 mg	125.0%	Carbohydrate	516.6 Gm	142.0%
Pyridoxine B_6	5.539 mg	276.0%	Weight	4366 Gm	n/a
Cobalamin B_{12}	0.0 Ug	0.0%	Dietary Fiber	88.41 Gm	304.0%

Percent of calories from: Protein: 13% Carbohydrate: 79% Fat: 8%

This chart shows that the sample daily menu on page 55 for a healthy, active male, age 25 to 50, is more than adequate!

Only you can decide if you want to make immediate changes, or if you prefer to make changes gradually.

← ***Key idea!***

To be successful in dietary transition, you must create your own natural environment as much as possible. The most important place to start is your home. Don't bring fats, oils, salt, sugar, processed foods, or animal

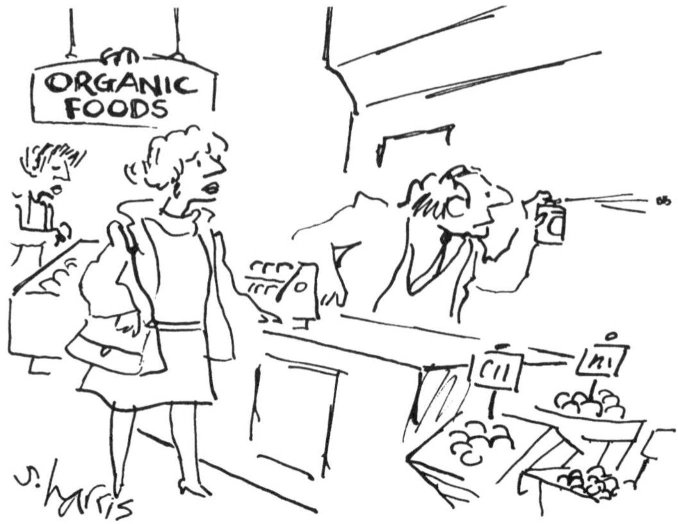

products into your home—not even "just for company." If you have these temptations around, you will either give in to them or waste a lot of energy resisting them.

Menu and recipe ideas to help you get started

The bottom line is that what you should be eating—meal after meal, day after day, for *life*—is a wide variety of fresh fruits and vegetables, steamed vegetables, and cooked starches (such as potatoes, yams, hard squashes, brown rice, millet, and quinoa). Small servings of naturally rich, high-fat vegetable foods—such as raw, unsalted nuts and avocados—also can be used in moderation.

The most important thing to keep in mind is that you should eat large enough portions of food to meet your caloric needs. You also need to be careful not to eat so much fruit, nuts, and avocados that you end up trading in a high-sugar, high-fat, conventional diet for a high-sugar, high-fat, "natural" diet.

If you are just starting out, you may want to prepare these foods in a way that mimics your more familiar recipes—soups, stews, and casseroles. There are many recipe books available from the American Natural Hygiene Society that will help you.

As you get more experienced, you'll probably simplify your food preparation quite a bit. After all, the more time you spend playing around in the kitchen, the less time you will have to play everywhere else. You'll have more time to enjoy the great outdoors—hiking, canoeing, playing sports, and gardening; and the great indoors—reading great books, writing love poems, painting and drawing, making clothes, and, of course, creating the next generation of healthy children! ← ***Key idea!***

Breakfast ideas

A breakfast made from fresh fruit, lettuce, and celery is a quick, easy, and delicious way to start the day. Be flexible with your fruit choices, based on what is ripe and available in the market. Fruit smoothies (blended fruits) are also fun. Cooked oatmeal with a few raisins is another good breakfast choice that adds variety and some welcome additional calories. Here are a few ideas.

- *Fresh Fruit Salad (such as bananas, apples, and strawberries), lettuce and celery, 1–2 oz. of almonds or sunflower seeds*
- *Orange Juice Smoothie (blend orange, banana, and kiwi), oatmeal with raisins*
- *Melon Salad Supreme (variety of melons and berries), lettuce and celery*
- *Deluxe Citrus Salad (variety of citrus fruit, berries, and kiwi), lettuce and celery, 1 oz. of raw, unsalted almonds or sunflower seeds*

Lunch ideas

Eat a large amount of fresh salad vegetables every day!

Eat a very big fresh vegetable salad every day at lunch. You can include all of your favorite vegetables—lettuce, celery, sweet peppers, broccoli, cauliflower, cucumber, tomato, jicama, carrots, beets, peas, cabbage, and more! You can assemble a different combination each day for variety. Add to this the Tomato Avocado Dressing listed below (or better ones that you make up!), and you have the beginnings of a feast. In addition to your salad, have a large plate of steamed vegetables, plus a baked potato, or a bowl of soup. Here are some ideas.

- *Large vegetable salad, dressing, steamed vegetables, baked potato*
- *Carrot juice, large vegetable salad, dressing, Potato-Vegetable Soup, brown rice*
- *Corn on the cob, large vegetable salad, dressing, steamed vegetables*
- *Mixed vegetable juice, large vegetable salad, dressing, steamed vegetables, baked potato*
- *Large vegetable salad, dressing, steamed vegetables, steamed quinoa*

Dinner ideas

Dinner also begins with a fresh vegetable salad (or mixed vegetable platter), along with a healthful salad dressing or a little lemon juice. Follow this with a helping of rice and steamed vegetables, a hearty soup, or a tasty casserole.

Here are some sample dinner ideas.

- *Large vegetable salad, dressing, Brown Rice-Lentil Stew*
- *Mixed vegetable platter, dressing, steamed vegetables, Split Pea-Yam Soup over brown rice*

- *Vegetable salad, dressing, steamed vegetables, baked potatoes*
- *Vegetable salad, dressing, Potato-Vegetable Soup, Brown Rice-Lentil Stew*

Recipes

Delicious transitional recipes to help you get started!

The following recipes are intended to give you a starting point for making the transition to a healthful diet. Don't be afraid to come up with your own variations!

Tomato Avocado Dressing

1/2 tomato, diced; 1 avocado, peeled and sliced
1/2 cup celery juice or water; 8 basil leaves

Place all ingredients in a blender or food processor and puree until smooth. Serve immediately.

Brown Rice-Lentil Stew

4 cups lentils; 6 cups water; 2 cups celery juice
3 carrots, diced; 4 ribs celery, diced
3 tomatoes, diced; 1 red bell pepper, diced
1 sweet potato, peeled and diced
1 bunch spinach; 2 cups brown rice
2 cups water

Bring 2 cups of water to a boil; stir in rice. When the water comes back to a vigorous boil, put lid on pan and turn heat down to a very low setting, approximately 15-20 minutes. In an 8-quart soup pot, bring all the other ingredients to a boil. Reduce the heat to medium-low and simmer for 45 minutes. Mix rice with vegetables to serve.

Potato-Vegetable Soup

3 russet potatoes, peeled
1 large Yukon Gold potato
1 large yam, peeled; 3 ribs celery; 1/4 head cabbage
2 large rutabagas, peeled
10 button mushrooms, washed (optional)
Water or soup stock as needed

In a food processor or by hand, slice all of the ingredients and place in an 8-quart soup pot. Cover the vegetables with the liquid. For added flavor, add 3-4 cups of leftover steamed vegetables, chopped. Bring to a boil, then simmer for 40 minutes, or until all vegetables are tender. Blend in food processor, and serve.

Split Pea–Yam Soup
9 cups soup stock; 2 cups dry split peas
3 large yams and 2 potatoes, peeled and diced
3 ribs celery, diced
1 yellow onion, chopped or 1 Tbsp. dried flakes
1 tsp. dill; 1 Tbsp. garlic powder (optional)
1/2 tsp. oregano; 1/2 tsp. thyme; 2 bay leaves
Bring the soup stock or water and peas to a boil while preparing the other ingredients. Add the yams and potatoes and simmer for 30 minutes, stirring occasionally. Add the celery, onion, and spices and simmer until peas are tender (about 30 minutes more). Remove the bay leaves. If a smooth texture is desired, blend in a food processor until smooth.

▼ ▼ ▼ ▼ ▼

In the next chapter, you will learn how to get started on your new healthful diet.

6

Getting Started

The Natural Hygiene diet is a system of guiding principles to help you maximize your health potential, not an endless list of "do's and don'ts." In fact, it is somewhat of a mistake to refer to *the* Natural Hygiene diet, because that would suggest that there is *one* specific, inflexible, and stereotyped diet that fits *everyone.* Nothing could be farther from the truth. The Natural Hygiene diet always must be adapted to the needs of the individual person, not the other way around.

Since virtually every family and every culture include unhealthful eating habits in their customs and traditions, don't feel like you have to change your eating habits overnight. Don't get discouraged. Successful, permanent, and healthful change takes time, knowledge, and experience. There is an art to living healthfully in a world that is not always ready for change. ← ***Key idea!***

Eventually, you will achieve complete self-mastery when it comes to food! You will know when to eat, what to eat, how to eat, and when to stop. You will be at your ideal weight and will love how you feel. But, just like any other art, eating healthfully takes practice. You can't achieve the ideal instantly. The only thing you can do instantly is to make the commitment to change. The actual changing takes time and practice.

Take one step at a time!

The best way to succeed is to take one manageable step at a time, marching at a steady pace in the right direction. Don't put unrealistic expectations on yourself.

Fortunately, small changes can make a big difference. The most important step for most people—and in some ways the easiest—is to begin eliminating all animal products from your diet. No other single step can bring so much benefit. Read labels carefully to see if the item contains animal products (or any other ingredients you no

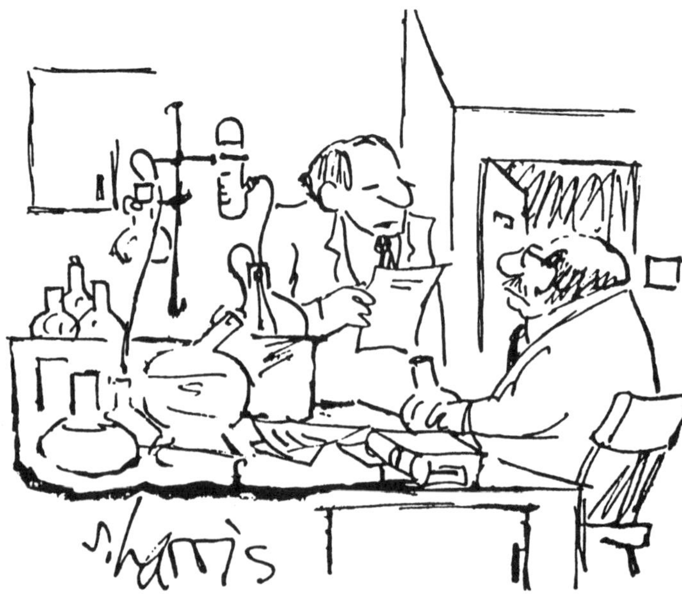

"Krantz, you are being awarded the Dugwell Prize for diligently working on one problem for 25 years without coming up with anything."

longer wish to include in your diet). Another very important step you can take right away is to start adding large portions of fresh fruit and vegetables to each day's menu, regardless of what else you eat.

Taking the plunge

Great tips to help you get started!

Changing your diet actually can be fun. It all starts in the kitchen, the one place where you have total control. Here are some tips to help you get started.

1. *Clean house.* Empty the refrigerator and cupboard of all the foods and condiments that are no longer on your menu. Many people start by getting rid of flour, coffee, sugar, salt and pepper, salad dressings, condiments (such as catsup and mustard), and a variety of other items.
2. *Keep healthful food on hand.* When you are hungry, you will go for whatever food is available. Stock your refrigerator with fresh fruits and vegetables; raw, unsalted nut butters for making salad dressings; and unsalted rice cakes or salt-free pita bread.
3. *Be sure to eat enough!* Fresh fruits and vegetables are low in calories. Add enough steamed vegetables, potatoes, legumes, and grains to ensure that you maintain reasonable weight and energy levels.
4. *Reinforce your new habits.* Give yourself plenty of credit for each positive step you take. Focus on your long-term goals rather than any little setbacks that can become excuses to "give up" too soon!
5. *Stay focused on the reasons for your new diet.* Eating more healthfully is not an end in itself. Good health only has meaning if you use it to have a great life. Discover what gives your life meaning. Become

all you can be and lead a wonderful life!

6. *Don't try to convert everyone else while you are just learning yourself.* It is natural to want to share new experiences with family and friends. But don't continually draw attention to the differences between you and the barbarians you live with (just kidding!). If you set a good example, and people see how much you are enjoying yourself, they will come to you to ask questions. Give them the same advice we are giving you—go one step at a time.
7. *Enjoy yourself.* The wonderful sense of well-being that comes with healthful eating is unbeatable! Don't miss it! Start improving your diet today—you are worth the effort!

First things first

As mentioned earlier, it is important to keep the big picture in mind when you start making dietary changes. Focus your attention on implementing changes in *your* diet and meal planning. Don't make the common mistake of trying to become an "instant expert" on diet and nutrition, and lecturing family and friends on how *they* should change *their* diets.

The most important first step! ➡

Remember, the most important step *you* can take to improve *your* diet is to eliminate or dramatically reduce your consumption of animal products—meat, fish, fowl, eggs, and dairy products. No other dietary change can produce such extraordinary benefits. Eliminate animal products from your diet *now.*

Later on, as you become more proficient in your new approach to eating (and show some of the benefits—such as increased energy, trimmer body, and overall bet-

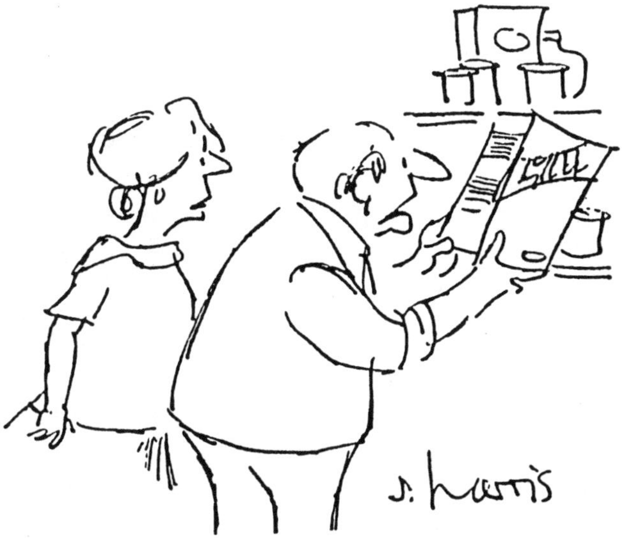

"Apparently some of the additives cause a nerve disorder, but some of the other additives cure it."

ter health), you will automatically begin to influence your loved ones. They will want those benefits, too!

Giving yourself credit for progress

People progress at different rates. Don't compare yourself to others who are farther along the path of change than you are. Move forward at your own pace—and make the choices that are best for *you.*

Give yourself credit for each step you take, even if you think it is just a little one. This is very important if you are going to continue to make healthful changes in your eating habits.

Living in the real world

We all live in the real world, with its temptations and seductions. It is important to develop your own set of strategies to support a healthful diet and lifestyle. It is also important to review these strategies, as well as your reasons for wanting to live healthfully.

Get as many tools as you can—books, cassette tapes, and videos—and use them, over and over, to bolster your decision to adopt a more healthful diet. Attend American Natural Hygiene Society conferences and seminars periodically—to learn new information and to reinforce your health-promoting habits. Cultivate friends who value their health and happiness. Pursue activities and interests that give you a feeling of productivity and emotional nourishment rather than looking solely to food to make you feel good.

Remember, one of the most important concepts that you will ever learn about diet and nutrition is that food is *fuel.* It is so very important that you eat to live and not live to eat.

▼ ▼ ▼ ▼ ▼

In the next chapter, you will learn how to make some very delicious and healthful recipes.

7

Sample Recipes and Food Tips

The Natural Hygiene diet is extraordinarily flexible and, with a little practice, easy to implement and enjoy! Once you master your understanding of the major principles, you will be well on your way to receiving the wonderful benefits.

The most important concepts are:

1. ***Base your diet primarily on fresh, uncooked fruits and vegetables.***
2. ***Eliminate or dramatically reduce your consumption of animal products—meat, poultry, fish, eggs, and dairy products.***
3. ***Become aware that food is merely delightful fuel, and not a form of entertainment.***
4. ***Simplify your meals as much as possible.***
5. ***Eat when you are genuinely hungry.***
6. ***Eat enough food to maintain your weight and energy levels.***
7. ***Don't overeat.***

You have an amazingly wide range of foods to choose from. There are countless varieties of fresh fruits; veg-

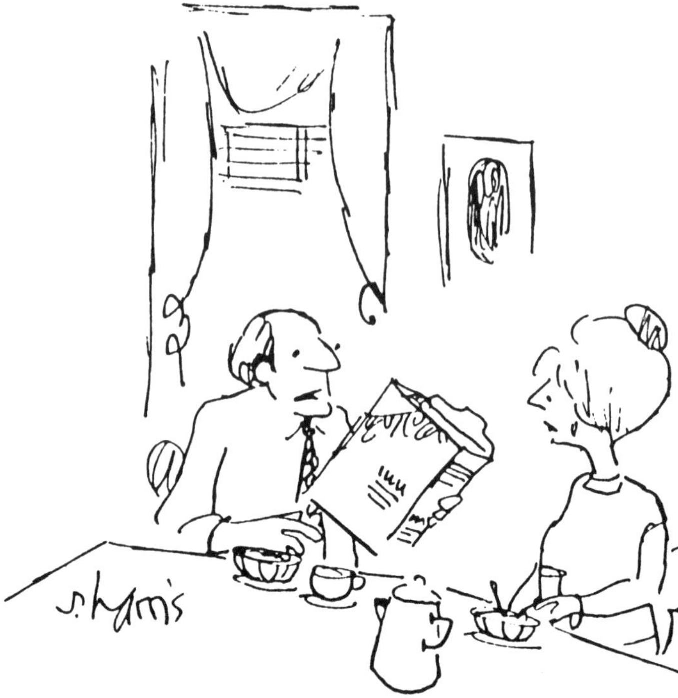

"One four-ounce serving supplies the minimum daily requirement of butylated hydroxyanisole, ethyl acetate, propylene glycol, ferrous lactate..."

etables; potatoes and hard squashes; whole grains and legumes; and raw, unsalted nuts and seeds. Prepare yourself for a delightful taste adventure as you explore your new way of eating! (See page 52.)

Remember, people come in all shapes, sizes, metabolisms, heights, weights, and ages. We each also have individual digestive capacities. That is why you need to fashion a diet that meets *your* individual needs.

Those who have followed the Natural Hygiene approach to diet for decades tend to eat amazingly simple meals, with hardly a thought given to elaborate meal preparation, or even regular mealtimes. When they get hungry, they eat the freshest fruits and vegetables in season, adding enough concentrated foods, such as lightly steamed vegetables, legumes, and cooked starches (such as potatoes, yams, hard squashes, and brown rice), and small servings of raw, unsalted nuts and avocados.

If these folks are not hungry, they skip a meal or two until they get hungry again. They have truly transcended the "three square meals," "meat and potatoes," "It's time for dinner," "Clean your plate," "I made it especially for you," approaches to eating. They are liberated.

But it takes time, experience, and a dramatic self-confidence to swim strongly like they do against the tide of family and social pressures, not to mention the years of bad eating habits that hold most of us back.

Fortunately, you don't have to jump into those deep waters to get tremendous benefits. Relatively modest first efforts will bring about amazing changes.

A week of health-supporting menus

Here is a one-week sample menu that draws upon a number of great recipes that appeared in *Health Science* magazine. Recipes follow the suggested menus.

Monday

Breakfast:
Fresh Fruit Salad, celery, and one ounce each of almonds and raw pumpkin seeds

Lunch:
Tossed Salad with Avocado Tomato Dressing, huge plate of steamed vegetables, and baked potato

Dinner:
Raw Vegetable Platter, Steamed Vegetable Medley, and Lentil Stew with Brown Rice

Tuesday

Breakfast:
Orange Juice Smoothie, Oatmeal with Raisins

Lunch:
Raw Vegetable Platter with Avocado Dip, steamed vegetables, and Sweet Potato Yam Soup

Dinner:
Fresh Green Salad, Cucumber Avocado Dressing, plate of steamed vegetables, and Split Pea Soup over Brown Rice

Wednesday

Breakfast:
Melon Salad Supreme or Pineapple Deluxe with lettuce and celery

Lunch:
Spring Salad, Spring Vegetable Soup, and baked potato

Dinner:
Tossed Salad with Broccoli Tahini Sauce, Stuffed Red Peppers, and Millet Squash Casserole

Thursday

Breakfast:
Fresh Fruit Salad, lettuce, and one ounce each of raw, unsalted almonds or sunflower seeds

Lunch:
Tossed Salad, Citrus Dressing, Steamed Vegetable Medley

Dinner:
Raw Vegetable Platter, Avocado Celery Dressing, Golden Parsnip Soup, and Broccoli and Cauliflower Casserole

Friday

Breakfast:
Deluxe Citrus Salad, lettuce and celery, and one ounce each of raw, unsalted almonds or sunflower seeds

Lunch:
Salad Potpourri and Minestrone Dinner Soup

Dinner:
Spring Salad, Summery Avocado Soup, and Vegetable Rice Casserole

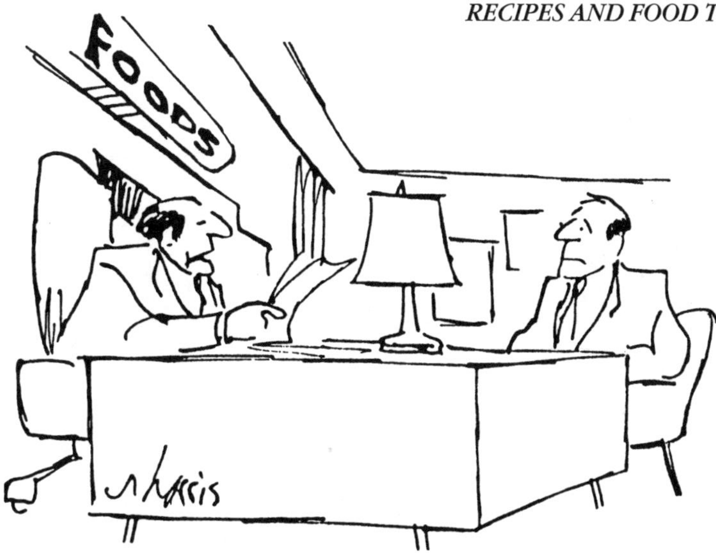

"Well, since they found excessive amounts of insecticide in our long-grain rice, let's repackage it and sell it as long-grain insecticide."

Saturday

Breakfast:
Fresh Fruit Smoothie and Oatmeal with Raisins

Lunch:
New Year's Salad with Steamed Artichoke Platter

Dinner:
Tossed Salad, Crunchy Avocado Dressing, Eggplant with Tomato Sauce, baked potato or brown rice

Sunday

Breakfast:
Fresh Fruit Platter, lettuce and celery, and one ounce each of almonds and raw pumpkin seeds

Lunch:
Peerless Potato Salad, Steamed Vegetables, and Tomato Zucchini Soup

Dinner:
Fresh Green Salad, Avocado Tomato Dressing, and Squash Casserole with Brown Rice

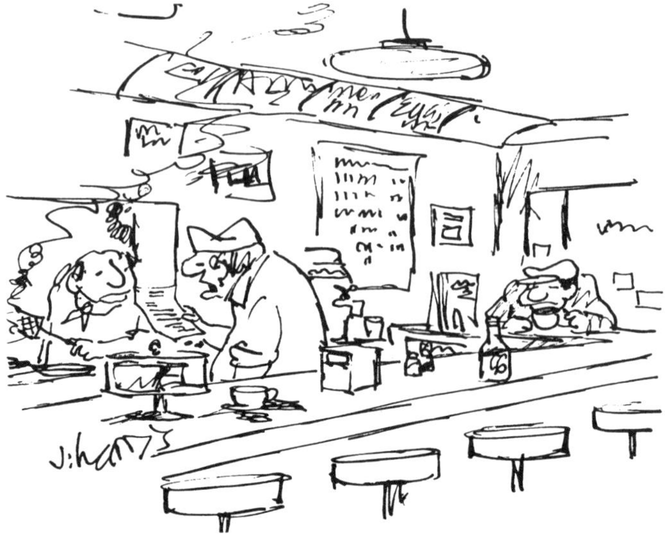

"We may be in trouble—the environmentalists have cited us as a hazardous waste site."

Enjoy these delicious recipes

The following recipes are great tasting and easy to make. There are no magical ingredients. If you can't find a particular fruit or vegetable, substitute for a similar one. Part of the joy of the Natural Hygiene diet is being flexible and creative. Because some of the recipes are simple fruit and vegetable salads, we have only listed the more elaborate recipes from the weekly menu. (Four recipes appear on pages 61-62.) *Bon appetit!*

Recipes

Fresh Fruit Salad

2 bananas, 2 apples, 1 cup strawberries

Tossed Salad

Leaf lettuce, carrot, beet, tomato, fresh green peas, cucumber, and alfalfa sprouts

Avocado Tomato Dressing

1 ripe avocado, 1 tomato, distilled water

Put avocado and tomato in a blender with just enough distilled water to keep the blade from sticking.

Raw Vegetable Platter

Carrots, jicama, celery, cucumber, alfalfa sprouts

Steamed Vegetable Medley

1 head of broccoli, 1 head of cauliflower, 4 summer squash, 1 stalk celery

Wash and cut vegetables into suitable sizes and steam for 5-7 minutes, depending on desired softness (or crunchiness).

Lentil Stew

2 cups dry lentils, 4-6 cups distilled water, 2 carrots (diced), 2 stalks celery (diced), 2 medium tomatoes (diced), small amount of green onion, leek, or chives, diced (optional), oregano or other herbs to taste

In a large kettle, bring 4 cups of water to boil. Add the lentils and remaining ingredients, cover, and turn the heat down to a low setting. Allow the lentils to cook for approximately 30 minutes. Check the water level frequently. It may be necessary to add water as the lentils swell.

Orange Juice Smoothie

1-2 cups orange juice (freshly squeezed if possible), 1 banana, 2 kiwi fruit

Blend until smooth. Serves one.

Avocado Dip

1 ripe avocado, 1 stalk celery, 1/2 large sweet red pepper, distilled water

Blend ingredients together in blender with just enough distilled water for desired consistency. Serve immediately.

Cucumber Avocado Dressing

2 large cucumbers, 1 large or 2 small avocados

Blend entire mixture until smooth. Serve immediately.

Split Pea Soup

2 cups split peas, 7 cups vegetable stock, 1 butternut squash

or yam (peeled and chopped coarsely), 2 large potatoes (diced medium), 2 large carrots (diced medium), 2 stalks celery (diced medium), 2 tsp. garlic powder (optional)
Simmer all the ingredients until the peas are tender, about one hour. Puree 1/3 of the mixture and return it to the pot. Simmer to desired temperature, and serve.

Spring Salad
Romaine, Bibb or red leaf lettuce; green or purple cabbage; cucumbers; celery; alfalfa sprouts; red peppers; broccoli; cauliflower

Spring Vegetable Soup
4 brussels sprouts, 2 carrots, 2 potatoes, 2 stalks celery, 6 stalks asparagus, vegetable stock
Prepare vegetable stock ahead of time (see recipe on p. 77). Cut ingredients into small bite-sized pieces. Steam for approximately 10 minutes. (Do not overcook.) Add asparagus during the last

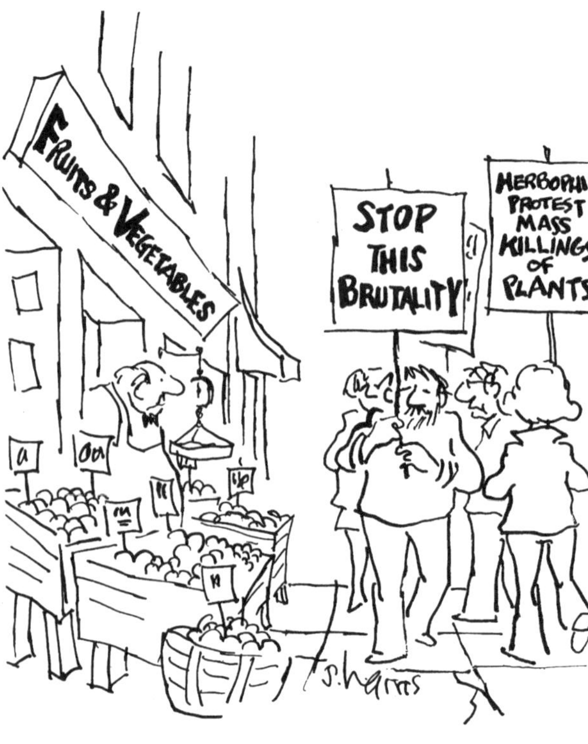
FRUITS & VEGETABLES
STOP THIS BRUTALITY
HERBOPHILES PROTEST MASS KILLINGS OF PLANTS
S. Harris

two minutes of steaming. Add steamed vegetables to vegetable stock and stir together.

Vegetable Stock

3 white turnips, 4 stalks celery, 2 large carrots

Clean and chop vegetables. Put in a pot, cover with water about 2 inches above vegetable level, and boil 20 minutes with the pot covered. Add nothing else. Let the vegetables cool for 30 minutes. Strain out broth. Blend the vegetables separately and use as a sauce over rice or other grain.

Broccoli Tahini Sauce

1 bunch steamed broccoli; 2 Tbsp. raw, unsalted tahini; 2 Tbsp. distilled water

Blend ingredients until smooth.

Stuffed Red Peppers

1 red pepper per person; 1/2 cup celery, finely diced; 1 medium avocado, mashed; 2 cut up tomatoes; 1/2 sliced red pepper; 1 cup mixed sprouts

Mix ingredients well with mashed avocado. Cut off tops from peppers and stuff each one.

Millet Squash Casserole

1/2 cup millet, browned slightly (dry), 2 cups water, 4 strips sliced celery, 3 small sliced zucchini squash

Bring water to a boil and add browned millet; cook about 10 minutes. Add celery, squash, and more water if necessary and cook about 15 minutes more, until tender and all water absorbed.

Melon Salad Supreme

1 watermelon, 1 cantaloupe or Crenshaw melon, 1 honeydew melon, 1 casaba melon, 1 pint strawberries (optional)

You can freely mix the different varieties and arrange them in a watermelon. Add strawberries for garnish and color.

Pineapple Deluxe

1 pineapple, 1 cup strawberries, 4 kiwi fruit, almonds, pecans or sunflower seeds (optional)

Cut the pineapple into bite-sized chunks and place into two bowls. Garnish each bowl with strawberries and peeled slices (circles, not wedges) of kiwi fruit.

Citrus Dressing

2 Tbsp. cashew nut butter, orange juice

Blend together, adding enough orange juice to achieve the desired consistency.

Avocado Celery Dressing

1 large or 2 small avocados, 1/3 cup celery juice, 1 tsp. lemon or lime juice

Blend everything together at a low speed until you achieve the consistency that you want.

Golden Parsnip Soup

6 crookneck squash, 4 zucchini squash, 4-6 parsnips, 1/4-1/2 cup distilled water, fresh parsley and basil (optional)

Steam the squash in one pan, the parsnips in another since they require different lengths of time. Steam until soft. Blend steamed squash with fresh herbs with enough water to make it "soupy." Pour most of the mixture into a large bowl. Add steamed parsnips a few at a time to the mixture in the blender, plus more water, if necessary, and blend until smooth. Pour into the bowl with the first batch of squash. Stir entire mixture together.

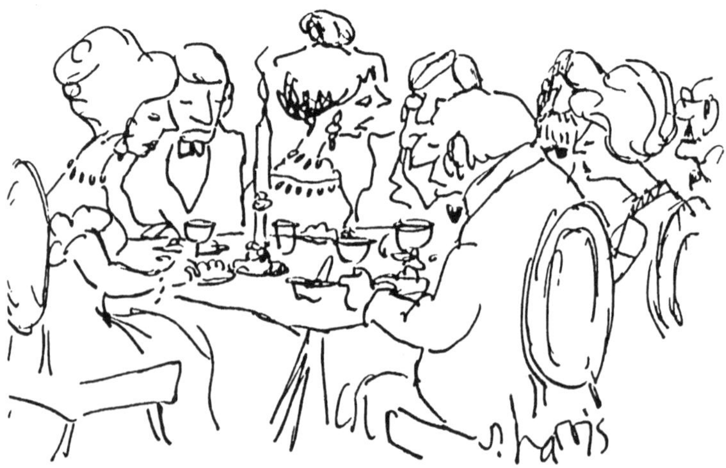

"I like the Pasteurs, but my goodness—
boiled tomato juice, boiled fish with boiled lettuce,
boiled bread and boiled butter, boiled salad..."

Broccoli and Cauliflower Casserole

1 cup cooked brown rice, 1 cup distilled water, 1 bunch broccoli, 1 head cauliflower, 4 stalks celery

While the rice is cooking, steam broccoli, cauliflower, and celery. Mix cooked rice and steamed vegetables together in a large bowl, or serve vegetables over rice in small serving bowls.

Deluxe Citrus Salad

4 oranges, 1 pineapple, 1 cup strawberries, 6 kiwi fruit, lettuce leaves

Peel or slice fruit, arrange on the lettuce leaves, eat, and enjoy.

Salad Potpourri

1 small head of broccoli, 1 small head of cauliflower, 1 red pepper, 1 cucumber, 1 medium tomato, 1/2 cup alfalfa sprouts, romaine lettuce

Cut and/or tear everything into bite-sized pieces. Mix it all together in a large bowl and serve as a tossed salad.

Minestrone Dinner Soup

10 cups stock or distilled water; 1 cup kidney beans; 1 cup garbanzo beans; 1 cup diced carrots; 1 cup diced celery; 1/2 cup diced green onions (optional); 3 cups peeled and diced tomatoes; 1 bunch spinach (chopped); 2 Tbsp. Italian herbs (optional); 1 Tbsp. garlic powder (optional); 1 cup whole wheat pasta or corn pasta

Place the washed beans in a large pot with 10 cups of stock (or water); boil for 2 minutes. Reduce heat and simmer 1-1/2 to 2 hours. Add carrots, celery, tomatoes, spinach, herbs, and garlic. Cover and simmer 45 minutes. Add pasta. Boil 10 minutes longer.

Summery Avocado Soup

4 summer squash, 4 zucchini, 1-2 ripe avocados

Lightly steam squash and zucchini. Blend steamed vegetables and avocado with enough of the water used in steaming until desired consistency is achieved.

Vegetable Rice Casserole

3 cups cooked brown rice, 1 cup peas, 2 cups diced carrots, 1 cup diced celery, 2 cups sliced green beans, 1 cup corn kernels, 1 tsp. thyme (optional), 2 cups vegetable stock

Combine rice, vegetables, and seasonings in a bowl. Place the mix in a covered casserole dish or loaf pan. Pour vegetable stock over the rice and vegetables until it just barely covers them. Bake at 350 degrees or until the carrots are tender.

Fresh Fruit Smoothie

1-2 cups organic apple juice (freshly made if possible), 1 banana, 2 kiwi fruit

Blend apple juice, banana, and peeled kiwi until smooth.

New Year's Salad

1 medium head of red leaf lettuce, 4 broccoli florets, 1 ripe sliced tomato, 1/2 sweet yellow pepper, 1/2 sweet red pepper, 1 stalk celery, raw cashews or almonds (optional)

Break the lettuce into bite-sized pieces into a bowl. Add tomato and slivered vegetables. Garnish with raw cashew nuts or almonds. Serves one.

Steamed Artichoke Platter

1 artichoke, 1/2 sweet red pepper, 1/4 cup snow peas, 6 brussels sprouts, 4 florets of broccoli, 4 florets of cauliflower, 4 baby carrots

Steam artichoke over boiling water for approximately 30 minutes. While the artichoke is cooking, steam the brussels sprouts in another pan. When the brussels sprouts are about half-way cooked, add the broccoli and cauliflower and steam for 5-7 additional minutes. Do not overcook! When the artichoke is cool enough to handle, cut out the center of the artichoke and fill with your favorite dressing. Arrange other vegetables around the artichoke.

Crunchy Avocado Dressing

2 large avocados, 2 stalks celery, 1 red pepper, distilled water

Dice the celery and red pepper and mix with mashed or blended avocado (blended with small amount of distilled water).

Eggplant with Tomato Sauce

1 diced eggplant; 10-12 large, ripe tomatoes (or 12 oz. tomato paste); 1 large diced bell pepper; 8-10 sliced mushrooms; small amount green onion, leek, or chives (optional); basil and/or oregano to taste

Cut the tomatoes into a large saucepan over low heat. Cover

and heat the pan for 3-5 minutes until the tomatoes begin to soften. Add the bell pepper, mushrooms, onion, herbs, and diced eggplant. The sauce should be the consistency of a thick soup. It may be necessary to add a small amount of water or a few tomatoes or a little tomato paste in order to get the desired consistency. Cook over low heat for approximately 30 minutes. Cooking time may vary, depending on the size of the eggplant chunks and on the low temperature setting. Stir frequently while cooking.

Fresh Fruit Platter

2 cups strawberries, 4 kiwi, 4 pears, romaine lettuce leaves
Wash, cut, and arrange fruit onto lettuce leaves.

Peerless Potato Salad

4 potatoes, lightly steamed; 1 small head of broccoli, steamed or raw; 4 stalks celery, diced; 2 avocados, mashed; romaine lettuce leaves
Wash and steam potatoes until tender. Cut into small pieces after cooling. Cut broccoli into small pieces or divide florets into individual pieces. Mix broccoli and diced celery with cut potatoes. Mash avocados and add to potato mixture.

Tomato Zucchini Soup

6-8 zucchini, 6-8 yellow squash, 3 tomatoes, fresh basil
Cut zucchini and yellow squash into 1-inch pieces and steam until soft but still a little crunchy. Cut tomatoes into quarters and blend until tomatoes become juice. Add diced basil. Continue blending until smooth. Gently mix tomato sauce with steamed squash.

Squash Casserole with Brown Rice

1 butternut squash, 2 cups cooked brown rice, 2 cups distilled water, 1 head cauliflower, 2 sweet red peppers
Bake butternut squash in 350 degree oven for approximately one hour, or until soft. Break cauliflower into small pieces and steam approximately five minutes. Cut red peppers into small pieces. Remove squash from oven, cut in half, and scoop out seeds. Remove skin if you don't want to eat it. Stir squash in with cooked rice. Mix steamed cauliflower and red peppers with the squash and rice.

Planning for success with your new diet!

Keep your meals simple and plan ahead. A little forethought can save you time and maximize your enjoyment of each meal. When you wash lettuce, wash enough for several meals. By planning a few meals ahead, you can save extra trips to the store at the last minute.

Begin your day with fruit for breakfast. Nothing could be simpler—or tastier! If you want more calories or just want the feeling of something more "substantial," make a breakfast of oatmeal and a few raisins.

At lunch, enjoy a fresh fruit salad or a tasty vegetable salad with natural dressing. Both of these choices will fill your appetite without filling you up. Add some salt-free rice cakes or crackers or salt-free pita bread if you are still hungry.

For dinner, start with a fresh salad. Add one of the great tasting dishes in this chapter. Try to eat at least several hours before you go to bed, and get up from the table right after eating.

Enjoy and savor each meal—but don't let your life revolve around what and when you are going to eat!

▼ ▼ ▼ ▼ ▼

In the next chapter, you will learn how to overcome some of the roadblocks to healthful eating.

8

Overcoming Roadblocks to Healthful Eating

The Natural Hygiene diet is delightfully easy to prepare at home. But what about when you have to go out to eat, or when you need to prepare food for guests who are coming to your house to eat? You may naturally feel some social pressure to "be like everybody else."

Some people thrive on being "different." But if you are like most people, feeling "different" can be very uncomfortable. In this chapter, you will learn some proven strategies to help you solve some of the family and social "situations" that are bound to arise when you start to eat healthfully.

Eating healthfully in the "real" world

Wouldn't it be great if all of our customs, traditions, laws, government agencies, and educational institutions supported a healthful diet? And, what if our parents and teachers taught us to eat healthfully from the time we were little children?

In this ideal setting, we could live just like our families, friends, and everybody else because it would be the healthy thing to do. We could "go along with the crowd" because the crowd would be on the right track.

But we don't live in an ideal world. We live in a world where traditions, folklore, culture, and customs lead not to the healthful life we all want, but to the pain, suffering, and sorrow of illness, and to premature death, for a great many people. That is why we need to reject many of the popular dietary practices of our time.

It is not possible to say with absolute certainty that the Natural Hygiene diet is the *ultimate* diet. It is merely the one most supported by current science. If you want the best available diet for yourself and your family, the Natural Hygiene diet is the one for you ...even if it makes a few waves around the dinner table.

Keeping answers simple

Key idea! ➨ It may be harder to talk effectively about the Natural Hygiene diet than it is to eat it. One good rule to follow is: *Don't talk about it too much at first.* If you are new to the Natural Hygiene diet and the occasion calls for you to say something about it, keep your comments short, simple, and honest. Say you are "trying it," or that you are "experimenting."

If you were to ask someone why they were eating an ice cream sundae, they most likely would say, "I like it." Or, "It tastes so good." These can be the same answers you give when you are asked about your new favorite foods and recipes. You don't have to be a walking encyclopedia of nutritional expertise.

You wouldn't expect to become an overnight expert

in car repair, carpentry, or chemistry. Don't feel like you need to become an instant expert on diet and nutrition. Often, the best approach is to become a picture of health, happiness, and good cheer.

Knowing what to say and *when* to say it is the first step in good communication. Thanksgiving dinner is *not* the time to lecture your relatives about their eating and drinking habits.

Strategies for successful interaction

Here are some tips to help you with friends and family as you begin to make healthful dietary changes.

1. Be yourself. The only person you have to convince

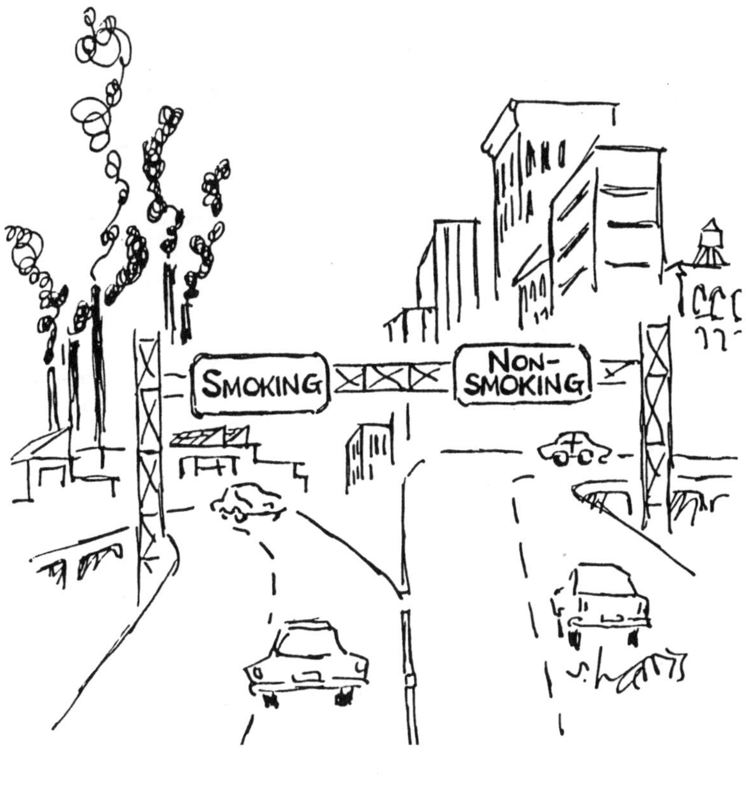

is you. You have a right to experiment. And you don't have to convince anybody else to try it.

2. *Be honest.* If people ask questions you can't answer, don't be afraid to say, "I don't know." You don't have to pretend to know more than you do.
3. *Pick your spots.* You don't have to give a lecture every time you go out to dinner. Timing is important. Before embarking on a long lecture to friends, be sure that they have a genuine interest.

Understanding your natural psychology

In addition to the strategies you need to address the potential obstacles you face when interacting with family and friends, you need to be prepared to deal with some mod-

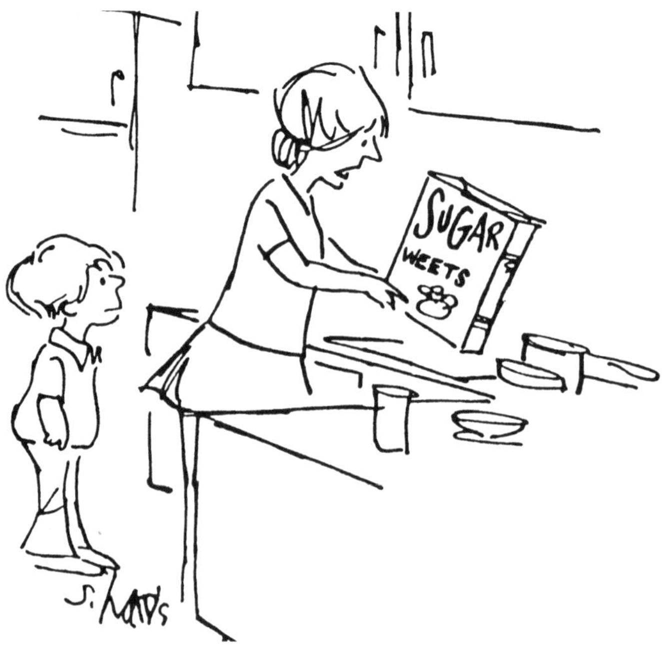

"...which is a special new preservative which keeps the food coloring from spoiling."

ern problems that can trick your natural psychology!

Have you ever made a New Year's resolution and then not pursued it? Psychologists have found that if a goal is too much trouble—even just a little bit too much trouble, you often won't pursue it. This is true even if you feel the goal is worthwhile!

Understand your natural history!

Doing what comes easiest has natural incentives. In the natural environment, animals constantly have to strive to get the "most" for the "least." Natural selection has gradually shaped these motivational mechanisms with remarkable precision.

For example, it is costly for a predator to make an energy investment mistake, such as attacking a strong animal when weaker prey is available. Predators' natural motivational systems usually facilitate good choices—helping predators to get the most energy (calories) for the least possible effort. This is a broad motivational principle in animal life—what might be called the "motive of energy conservation."

The same principle holds for much of human choice and behavior. When facing the harsh, natural world, you better prefer the most energy-efficient solution to life's troubles; otherwise, survival is threatened. We see evidence of this preference for energy conservation in our own motivation today—like having a tendency toward enjoying high-caloric food more than lower-caloric food when it is available.

Think of the last time you faced a list of errands. Probably you tried—at least briefly—to organize those errands in a way to save as much time and energy as possible. "Of course," you might be thinking. "What could be more obvious?" Of course you should try to get the most for the least. Why shouldn't you? It is only natural—and wise.

At least, it used to be.

Our unnatural world

Getting food today is too easy for your health!

Times have changed. Today, our natural motivational mechanisms can get us into trouble because we no longer live in the natural environment! We live in a modern environment that makes it easy to make choices that were never present in the ancestral world.

When our ancestors ate, they could not consume 1,000 calories of concentrated and processed sugar, fat, and salt in just a few bites. To get substantial calories, they had to expend substantial efforts. Obtaining those calories took a lot of effort, as did chewing and swallowing. Many of our health problems today result from amazing levels of human "progress" in food production and processing. Today, when we seek "the most for the least," we often wind up with way too much for too little effort. A lot of our modern foods "go down easily"—for example, 232 calories in a small chocolate bar, 530 calories in a hamburger, or 1,200 calories in a pint of ice cream. A lot of energy "in" for not much energy expended.

Leveling the playing field

Key idea! ➡ When it comes to good health, two key goals are 1) to eat whole natural foods, and 2) to exercise regularly. But be warned: both of these positive goals require energy expenditures that most Americans can easily avoid! Therefore, it is hardly surprising that many of us have difficulty actually integrating these habits into our lives. In today's upside-down world, these goals often take more effort and energy than less healthful alternatives. As a result,

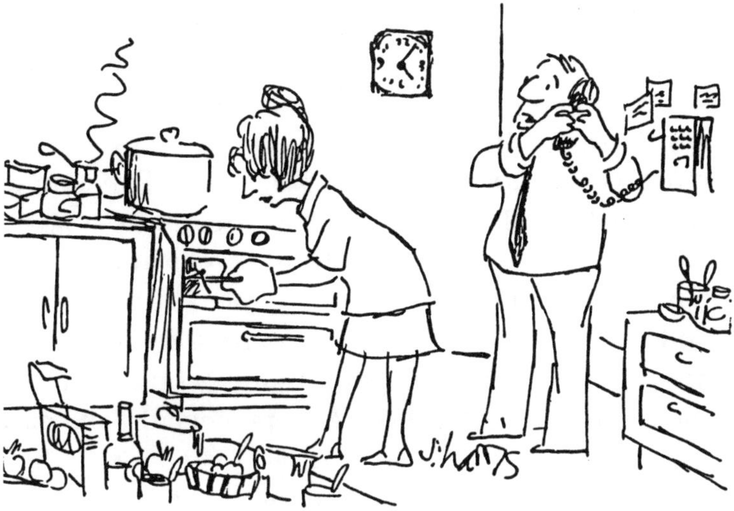

"Stop the presses. They're veggies!"

healthful habits can seem almost "unnatural"—and this is a potentially dangerous state of affairs.

If you have struggled with these issues, it may be time to rearrange some facets of your daily routine. The basic principle is to make healthful living as easy as possible—and unhealthful living as difficult as you can make it. In this way, you can "level the playing field" inside your psychology, giving healthful living a better chance of happening more consistently.

Strategies for healthful eating

Here are three strategies that many people have found useful:

1. Make sure that eating unhealthful foods is a serious hassle. You can accomplish this by following a simple behavioral rule: No junk food comes into your

house! This "no junk food" rule helps for two reasons. First, you won't have to deal with the stress of making the decision as to whether junk food comes home. It simply doesn't. The second helpful component is that getting unhealthful "treats" requires too much energy to bother with very often! This simple rule can help tilt the self-discipline odds in your favor.

2. Pack a lunch box with healthful snacks in the car. A "snack pack" of fresh fruits, dried fruits (such as raisins and dates), and nuts and seeds may help give your self-discipline a booster shot. Many people find that their most vulnerable hour occurs when driving past a grease distribution station (a fast-food outlet) when hungry, or even when not hungry. The snack pack can help you during these potentially weak moments.
3. Discover a mode of exercise that you find to be fun. Exercising goes against much of our natural energy-

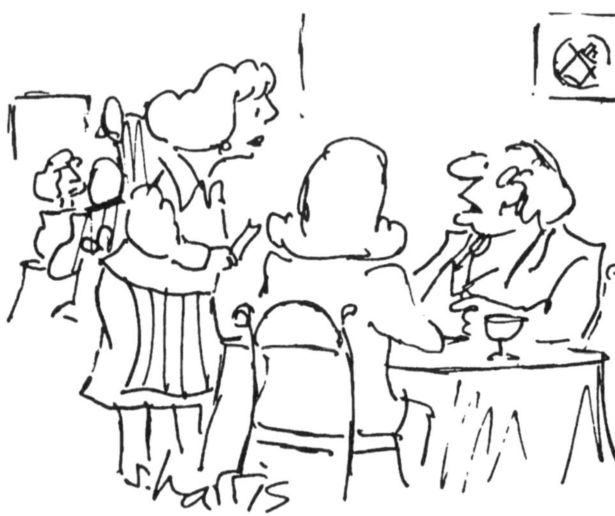

"Can we get caffeinated coffee in a no-smoking area?"

conservation programming. But, this is less true if we can find activities that serve a purpose. For some, that purpose may be the excitement of competition. For others, it may be the value of socializing with friends.

Enjoyment as a motivator

If you have started many exercise regimens in the past, only to quit after a short while, take heart! This may not be a sign of a lack of discipline on your part, but rather a lack of enjoyment for the activity. Exercise uses energy that we are designed to spend carefully, and grudgingly. Most of us will naturally resist expending this energy without good reason.

◀ Include fun in your health program!

Usually, "getting in shape" is not enough reason to sustain motivation. Having fun often is! Fun is sometimes needed to get us moving—and keep us going. So, experiment with yourself! Try new things—new ways of exercising! And consider adding a social element. If you and a friend establish a routine of walking together on Mondays, Wednesdays, and Fridays, then you both may be more likely to stick with it. For one thing, exercising with a friend can be more fun, so you want to do it. In addition, a regular routine can create subtle, but useful, social tension to aid your good intentions. It can become a hassle to not live up to your exercise/social obligation, which can be a very good thing.

Dangerous new world

Our modern world is a wonder of human genius and invention. Few of us would desire to rewind the clock of progress to a time when people routinely worked up to 80 hours per week at grueling physical labor just to survive. Most of our ancestors, ancient and recent, worked very hard simply to get enough calories—enough energy—to get by. They didn't need to "watch their waistlines," or to join a health club to "get in shape."

Generally speaking, we are better off today. But, our modern world has some dangerous conveniences—and our natural energy-conservation programming often can lead us astray. Easy access to unlimited quantities of rich foods—and work that requires minimal physical efforts—can compromise our health and well-being. Using our natural strategies of attempting to get "the most for the least" is no longer always the best way. Today, we have to be wise and determined—to put our energies in the right places—if we wish to enjoy the best possible results.

▼ ▼ ▼ ▼ ▼

In the next chapter, you will learn how to feed your children healthfully.

9

Feeding Healthy Children

Most people do not learn about the Natural Hygiene diet until they reach adulthood. How fortunate are the children whose parents feed them healthfully early in life—ideally, from birth.

It is truly a joyous experience to raise a child who is well nourished and not subjected to the unhealthful foods and beverages that most children eat and drink.

When designing a diet for your child, it is very important to realize that children are not little adults. Children are growing. They have faster heart beats, more rapid respiration, higher body temperatures, and faster metabolisms than do grownups. Adults have greater reserves with which to buffer their daily intake of nutrients than do children, and children need relatively more calories than adults.

Children have special needs!

Feeding your child: the first year

Breast milk should be the exclusive food for your child until at least the age of six months. Between six and eight months, the teeth begin to appear and the child naturally begins to reach for other foods on the table.

Cow's milk is the perfect food for baby cows.

Infants fed bottled cow's milk, or infant "formula" preparations, or cereals before the age of six months run the documented increased risks of respiratory, ear, and other infections; gastroenteritis; allergies; iron deficiency; anemia; and sudden infant death syndrome. They also run the risk of developing obesity, ulcerative colitis, coronary artery disease, and multiple sclerosis later in life.

Even after introducing other foods, breast milk should still provide 50% to 100% of the diet until one year of age, and 25% to 50% until age two.

Introducing new foods

After six months, and preferably after the child starts showing an interest in other foods, the child can be fed small amounts (one-two ozs.) of succulent, fresh, ripe fruit, with the seeds removed. These can be served either whole, chopped, or blended, depending on the number of teeth and the ability of the child to manage them. Use one fruit at a time, beginning once a day, and gradually increase the quantity and frequency up to three times per day.

Next, you can introduce succulent vegetables, such as cucumber and tomato, in small amounts. You also can feed your child blended fresh vegetables—such as romaine lettuce, celery, and green beans—at one to two meals per day. Add one vegetable at a time to the diet. If you wish, you may feed lightly steamed green and yellow vegetables and starches (such as squash and white and sweet potatoes) to your child once a day.

Raw, unsalted nuts such as almonds or cashews may

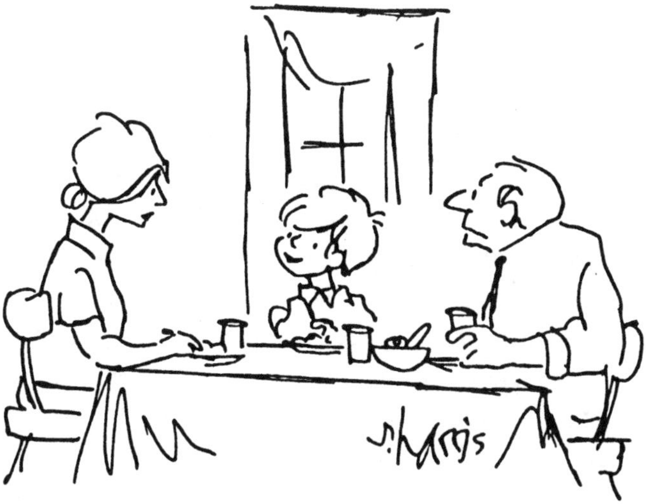

"But I'm not leaving it over—
I'm saving it for the compost pile."

be blended with water or fresh fruit juice to produce a nut "milk" or nut "cream." These can be fed by spoon or bottle, depending on consistency, one or two times a day. Some children may not gain the ideal amount of weight during their first year if their diet is too high in raw green vegetables, because these foods are low in calories and high in water and fiber. If your child falls in this category, add more nut milks or creams and/or steamed starches, and decrease the amount of raw vegetables in the diet. Cooked rice cereal also may be used occasionally.

Feeding your child: the second year

After one year of age, breast milk can still make up 25% to 50% of the child's diet until age two. In addition, your child can eat most raw fruits and vegetables; steamed green, yellow, and starchy vegetables; cooked whole grains and legumes; and some blended, raw, unsalted nuts and seeds that have been mixed with vegetables to ensure safety in swallowing.

The daily diet, until age two or three, should be:

- breast milk (one to four times per day);
- fresh fruit (one to two times per day);
- raw vegetables (one to two times per day);
- steamed vegetables (one time per day);
- cooked starchy vegetables (squash, corn, white and sweet potatoes) or whole grains, such as oatmeal, cornmeal, buckwheat, millet, brown rice, barley, and whole grain bread (one to two times per day);
- concentrated proteins in the form of raw, unsalted nuts or seeds and cooked legumes, such as lentils, beans, and peas (maximum one time per day).

Sample daily menus

Breakfast: fresh, ripe fruit; or whole grain cereal (add chopped fruit, nut milk or soy milk, if desired)

Snack: fresh fruit or raw vegetables

Lunch: raw vegetable salad, chopped or in small pieces (add avocado chopped or blended with tomato and celery as dressing if desired); or fresh, ripe fruit; or whole grain bread with avocado as a spread (optional); and a small handful of raw, unsalted nuts or seeds or nut butter (optional)

Dinner: raw vegetable salad, steamed vegetables, and cooked starchy vegetable or whole grain or cooked legume

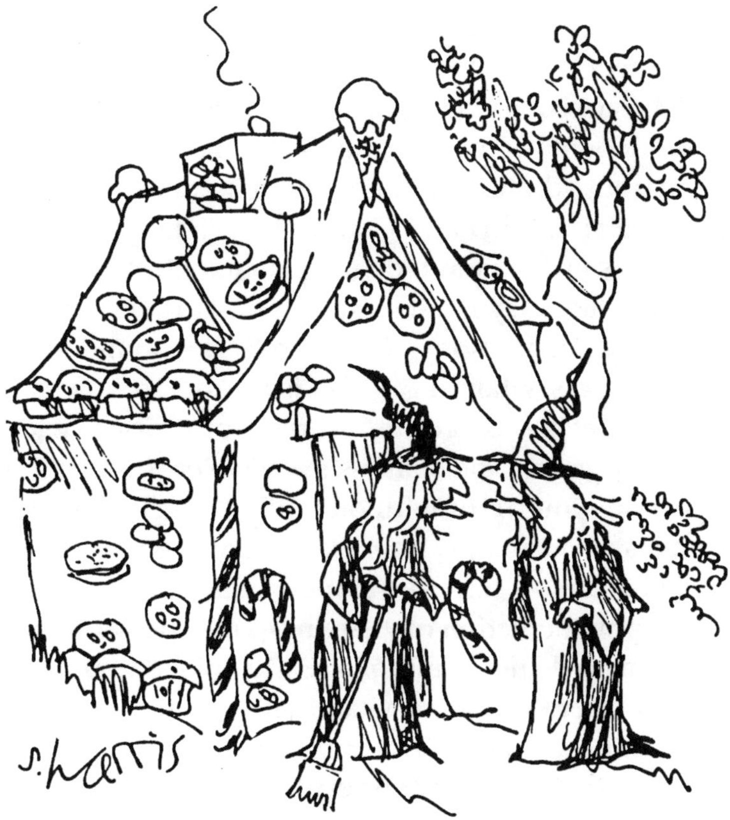

"You may not believe it, but it's made from a mix."

Age two and beyond

After the age of two, the only dietary changes are: decreasing and stopping breast milk and increasing the frequency of other foods.

Children do not need, nor should they have, any foods from animal sources. A balanced vegetarian diet is more than adequate for their needs. Serving them animal foods will put them at greater risk for developing diseases of the heart and blood vessels, kidneys, skin, and gastrointestinal tract, as well as arthritis, allergies, osteoporosis, and cancer.

A balanced vegetarian diet supplies more than adequate amounts of essential nutrients, including proteins, fats, carbohydrates, vitamins, and minerals. The exceptions are vitamin D and vitamin B_{12}. Vitamin D comes from the sun. If children do not get enough exposure to the sun, they may need to supplement their diet. The highest concentrations of vitamin B_{12} are found in animal products. Vitamin B_{12} also is synthesized in small amounts by bacteria on the surface of various vegetables, leafy greens, and some sea vegetables. Modern food processing interferes with our ability to get significant amounts of vitamin B_{12} from plant sources. Because some total vegetarians have developed vitamin B_{12} deficiencies, supplementation of vitamin B_{12} may be warranted. People who do not want to have their blood tested periodically to evaluate their vitamin B_{12} levels should consider taking a vitamin B_{12} supplement.

Your child deserves the very best. Children raised on a diet which excludes animal sources will not feel they are missing anything—so why not provide them with the best possible future health!

▼ ▼ ▼ ▼ ▼

In the next chapter, you will learn the latest thinking on the practice of food combining.

10

Food Combining Made Easier

The popular practice of food combining—eating simple meals with foods selected based on the concept of digestive compatibility—originated with Natural Hygiene.

Food combining found its greatest proponent in Dr. Herbert Shelton, one of the founders of the American Natural Hygiene Society, who published a little booklet titled *Food Combining Made Easy.* Dr. Shelton's practice as a physician brought him into contact with tens of thousands of people who had developed diseases that were reversible through the practice of Natural Hygiene, including dramatic dietary changes.

Through experience, Dr. Shelton discovered that his patients, especially those with eating disorders, such as compulsive overeating, could avoid the dietary excesses that had contributed to their ill health if they were very rigid in their eating habits.

In 1951, when Dr. Shelton first published *Food Combining Made Easy,* much less was known about nutrition and human physiology than is known today. Dr. Shelton hypothesized that indiscriminate combinations of foods, which he classified into categories (proteins, starches, fruits, and vegetables), were indigestible in the human stomach. To help his patients avoid "bad combinations" of foods, he devised a set of food combining rules, which are summarized in the following three recommendations:

1. *Don't eat concentrated proteins and concentrated starches at the same meal.*
2. *Don't eat fruit with either concentrated proteins or concentrated starches.*
3. *Vegetables can be eaten with either concentrated proteins or concentrated starches.*

Can aid in weight loss! ➡

Many people have become acquainted with the concept of food combining from reading about it in the best-selling book, *Fit For Life,* co-authored by Harvey Diamond and Marilyn Diamond. *Fit For Life* helped millions of people transform their eating habits, and many were delightfully surprised to find that, when they simplified their meals, they lost weight.

The real benefits of food combining

There is no scientific evidence to back up the assertion that we must eat only certain combinations of foods at a single meal or face dire consequences. But, everyone who has employed food combining successfully has enjoyed some very real benefits. Because they eat simpler meals, they are much less likely to overeat. The indigestion and other problems experienced when foods are "improperly combined" are more likely related to overeating (especially overeating on concentrated foods) and/or individual digestive limitations than anything that can reasonably be attributed to "bad food combining."

A new pattern of eating!

Most of us developed atrocious eating habits in early life and need to make dramatic changes if we want to be healthy. Food combining offers us a new pattern of eating, one that helps us make the transition to a healthful, plant-based diet, and helps us develop a new and healthier attitude toward eating.

One admonition of the old food combining rules still holds true—eat fruit as a meal by itself. Fresh fruit takes less time to make its way through our digestive tract

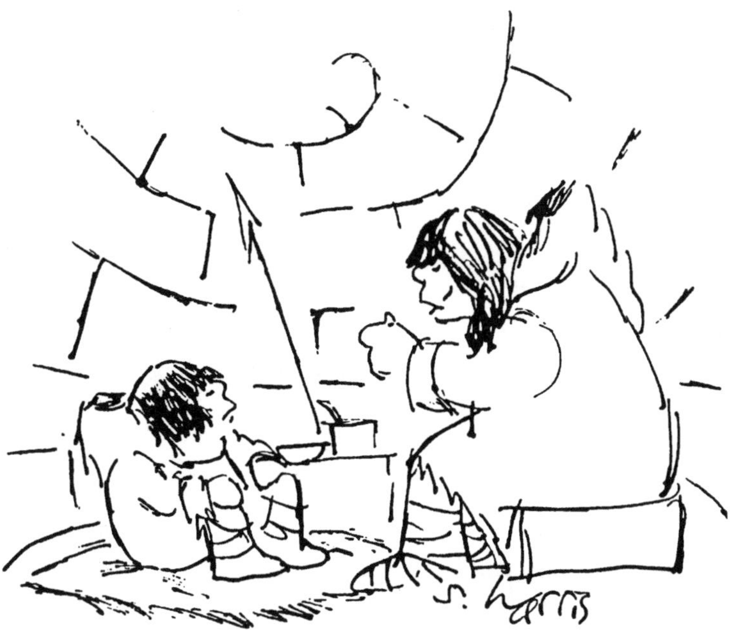

"Every day you should eat something from each of the five basic food groups: fried blubber, boiled blubber, stewed blubber, baked blubber, and raw blubber."

than other foods. So, if we eat fruit with foods that take longer to digest, they may not digest well.

Natural Hygiene diet

Research resoundingly supports the two central dietary recommendations of Natural Hygiene—eat a plant-based diet, and do not overeat. In addition, there are further benefits because 1) a large portion of the Natural Hygiene diet is uncooked, and 2) the emphasis is on vegetables, rather than grains, in contrast to other vegetarian diets. When these recommendations are adopted,

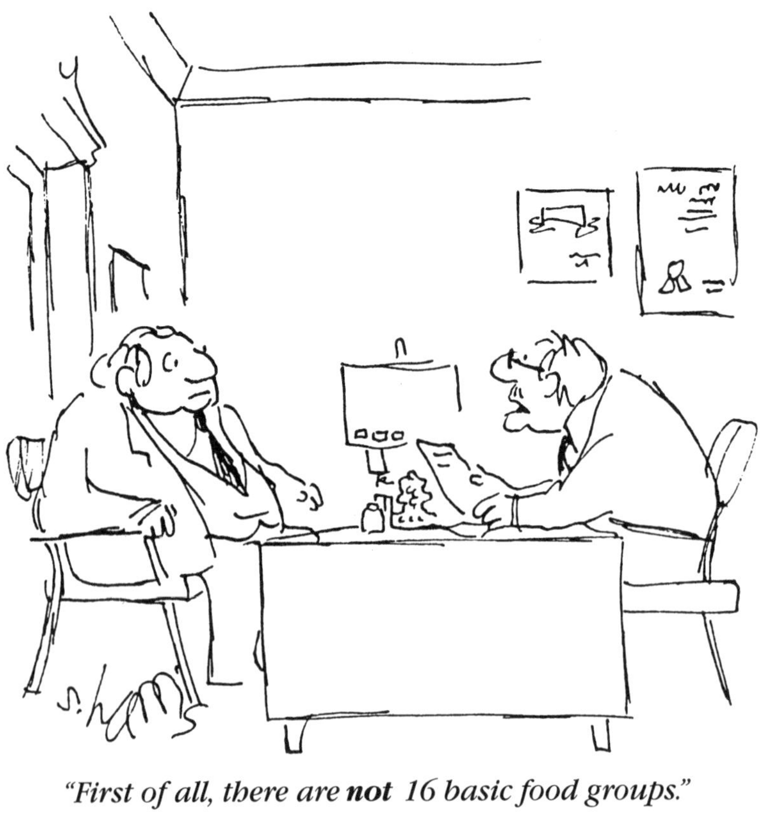

*"First of all, there are **not** 16 basic food groups."*

food combining offers little, if any, additional benefit.

For those people who are not yet willing or able to adopt the Natural Hygiene dietary recommendations, food combining may make a significant difference. Dr. Shelton targeted *Food Combining Made Easy* to just such an audience. He recognized that if people were going to eat meat, fish, poultry, eggs, and dairy products, they would be less likely to overeat if they were limited to just one of these "foods" at a meal. That way, they would not be eating as much concentrated food.

Dr. Shelton realized that it would help people even more if they avoided other concentrated foods, such as complex carbohydrates, when eating animal products. To a certain degree, food combining was an attempt to minimize the price people had to pay for eating foods that they should not have been eating in the first place.

Feeding children

Feeding your child a plant-based diet is much more important than food combining!

Food combining rules can be overly restrictive for children. Many growing children are picky eaters. Therefore, arbitrarily restricting the foods they eat can lead to problems. Members of the International Association of Hygienic Physicians report that they see many children whose well-meaning parents are trying to put rigid food combining practices above the primary Natural Hygiene food recommendation—to eat a wide variety of whole, natural, plant foods.

These physicians feel that it is wrong for parents to overemphasize food combining. Children are very peer-oriented. It is hard enough for them to forego the junk foods—burgers, soft drinks, pizza, candy, ice cream, etc.—their friends eat, without having to worry about food combining. Parents should be happy if their children are willing to eat whole, natural foods.

Natural Hygiene: the science of health

The benefits of Natural Hygiene are not linked to food combining.

People with digestive problems can benefit by simplifying their meals. However, food combining as a general admonition to the overall population is neither supported by science nor experience. Food combining is not a necessity for people who are eating healthful, plant-based diets. However, food combining can help curtail appetite. This may help people avoid overeating and help them keep their weight down.

The American Natural Hygiene Society and the IAHP still recommend that people eat simple, uncomplicated meals. Neither group is asking anyone to stop practicing food combining if it is helping them to live more healthfully. But both groups think that it is time for Natural Hygienists to focus less on food combining because it creates unnecessary stress for people. In addition, critics of Natural Hygiene have used food combining as evidence that Natural Hygiene is not based on science.

▼ ▼ ▼ ▼ ▼

In the next chapter, you will get answers to the most commonly asked dietary questions.

11

Frequently Asked Questions

Beginning a new diet can be like stepping into new territory. Even though you know the destination is well worth the effort, you may have questions as you set out on your journey.

The following are some of the most frequently asked questions by people who are attempting to make healthful dietary changes.

Is the Natural Hygiene diet an all-raw food diet?

No. There is no *one* diet that can meet everyone's needs at all times. The American Natural Hygiene Society recommends that people eat a diet derived exclusively from whole, natural foods—predominantly fresh fruits and vegetables, with the variable addition of nuts, legumes, and whole grains—matched to their individual needs and capabilities.

← ***Each of us has individual needs!***

It is this emphasis on raw, fresh fruits and vegetables that distinguishes the Natural Hygiene diet from other vegan diets, most of which emphasize cooked grains.

But while raw food *predominates* (by volume) in the Natural Hygiene diet, a *totally* raw-food diet it is not a requirement for health.

Furthermore, a diet that might be appropriate for an eighty-pound, eighty-year-old female may be substantially different from the diet for an active, 220-pound, twenty-year-old, male athlete. People who have colitis have limited digestive abilities. An older person who has no teeth will need to eat differently from a young, growing child.

Our allegiance must be to our individual needs, not to any philosophical or ideological concepts. Our needs can change over time, depending on our activity level, state of health, and the specific goals we are trying to accomplish.

The best diet you can have! ➠

The best diet is the one that enables us to meet our individual energy and nutrient needs, with the least amount of toxic load or other negative effects. For most people, that translates to a diet made up of a large volume of fresh, raw fruits and vegetables (which are the best source of vitamins, minerals, proteins, fat, water, and fiber); and enough concentrated foods (such as potatoes, yams, legumes, small quantities of raw, unsalted nuts, and whole grains) to meet our energy needs.

Will I get enough protein on a vegetarian diet?

Getting enough protein should not be a problem! ➠

Yes. A calorie-sufficient diet that includes a broad base of fresh fruits, vegetables (especially leafy greens, yellow vegetables, and cruciferous vegetables), a small amount of seeds and nuts, and complex starches (including potatoes, grains, and legumes) will provide the appropriate amounts of needed nutrients.

As a general guideline, a nutritional program that contains 10-15% total calories from unsaturated nut, seed, and plant-based fats and 10-15% protein (eliminating all animal and dairy products) is recommended.

Will I need to take vitamin and mineral supplements? No. When you eat a calorie-sufficient diet derived exclusively from whole natural foods—fresh fruits and vegetables, and the variable addition of whole grains, nuts, and legumes—you get an abundant supply of both the *quantity* and *quality* of vitamins your body needs. Vitamin B_{12} is a possible exception.

Vitamins are essential substances needed by the body to catalyze a variety of enzymatic and other functions. If an individual does not obtain the required quantities

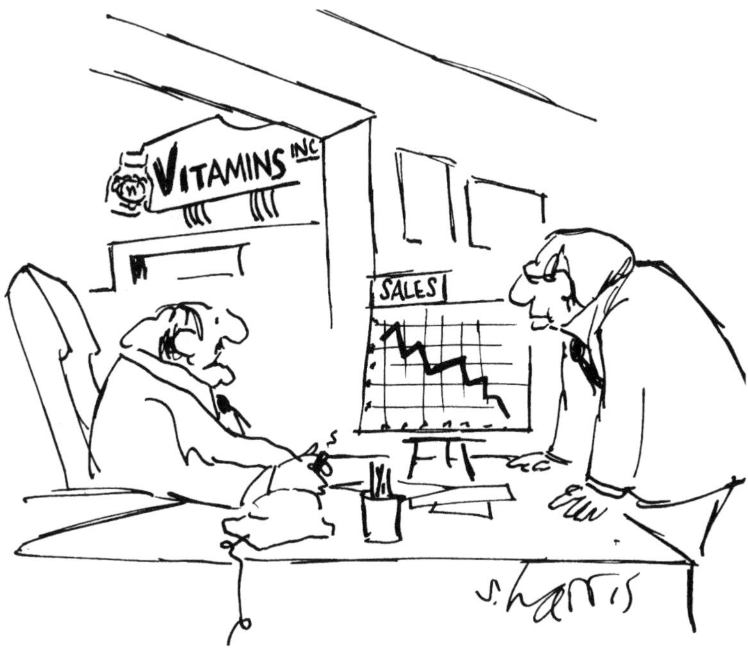

"Megavitamin therapy—that's the answer!"

of these nutrients, health may suffer. If the diet does not provide optimum levels, supplementation may provide some benefits, along with potential risks. If the diet provides the nutrients, supplementation may, in some circumstances, be harmful.

Will I get enough calcium on a Natural Hygiene diet to prevent osteoporosis?

Every natural plant food contains calcium. Vegetarian populations, even those with low calcium intake, have much lower rates of osteoporosis than older women in high-meat-eating countries.

The best prevention for osteoporosis is a low-protein diet with an abundance of fresh fruits and vegeta-

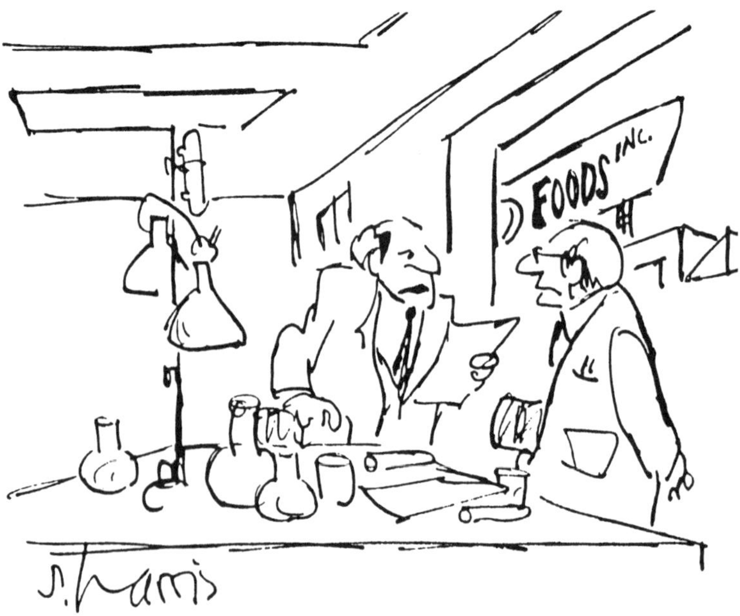

"Before we add any more preservatives, let's determine if it's worth preserving."

bles, especially green leafy vegetables, coupled with weight-bearing exercise.

How can I be assured of getting adequate vitamin B_{12} on a vegan (total vegetarian) diet?

Vitamin B_{12} exists in highest concentration in animal and dairy products. However, vitamin B_{12} also is synthesized by bacteria that live on the surface of various vegetables and leafy greens. It also can be found in sea vegetables and some yeast products.

Vitamin B_{12} plays an important role in the production of red blood cells and the integrity of the spinal cord. Although people on a vegan Natural Hygiene diet will often have lower blood levels of B_{12} than people on a conventional, meat and dairy diet, the lower levels apparently are sufficient to maintain red cell production and spinal cord health.

If you have been a vegan for more than three to five years, you should take a blood test once a year to evaluate your B_{12} level. Occasionally, people may develop a deficiency. Supplementation may be warranted. If your serum levels drop abnormally low, symptoms of neurological damage can occur and may be permanent.

Since the Natural Hygienie diet excludes table salt, would salt substitutes be acceptable?

A diet derived from fresh fruits, vegetables, and the variable addition of nuts, legumes, and whole grains—with the exclusion of animal foods, processed foods, and added salt—will be very low in sodium (about 500 mg. per day or less). This is more than enough to meet our bodily needs, but not enough to contribute to the many problems associated with excess salt intake, such as high blood pressure and edema (swelling).

A low-sodium diet also is less stimulating to the appetite; thus, you are much less likely to overeat on a low-sodium and low-spice diet. Salt substitutes often contain other substances, such as potassium chloride, which can taste like salt (sodium chloride). Unfortunately, these salt substitutes often have similar effects on the body in terms of blood pressure and appetite stimulation. Some of the "substitutes" are derived from dehydrated vegetables and have very high sodium levels, despite their "natural" label.

The best solution is to allow the body to develop a taste for less stimulating food by avoiding salts *and* their substitutes. If salt is to be used during a transition to healthful eating, it only should be put on the surface of the food—after cooking. This gives the most salt taste with the least amount of sodium. The less added salt or salt substitutes, the better.

Should we drink six to eight glasses of water daily? How much water—the American Natural Hygiene Society recommends distilled water—to drink each day depends entirely upon individual factors. If you eat a succulent, high-water-content diet, avoid table salt, and do not engage in strenuous physical activity, it is doubtful that you need to drink much additional water. However, in most cases it is better to err on the side of "too much" water, rather than too little. If you eat more cooked foods and concentrated foods, consume salt, and work out intensely, sweating profusely, you may need more than eight glasses per day.

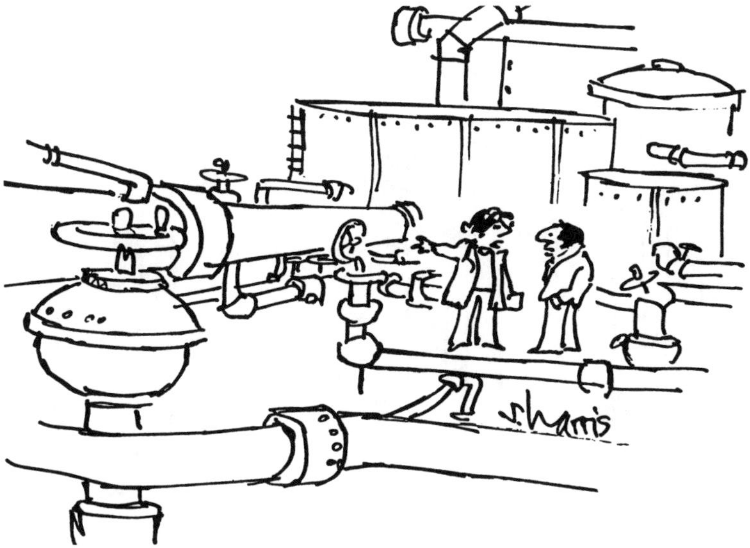

"By processing this seawater, we now can create 100,000 gallons of detergent-filled drinking water every day."

Does drinking with meals contribute to indigestion and intestinal gas? Do we get adequate water just from eating fresh fruits and vegetables?

It is possible that diluting your digestive juices may interfere with digestion. However, that does not mean you cannot drink with meals. If you expect to be extra thirsty, it is probably best to drink before your meal, preferably by ten to fifteen minutes.

Fruits and raw vegetables can provide all your fluid requirements when you eat a balanced vegetarian diet. Whether you have a juicy salad along with baked potatoes, or you drink some water with your potatoes, you are still having water with your meal—and that is normal and appropriate. However, when your fluid requirements are very high, such as when you are exercising in a hot environment, you have to make extra effort to in-

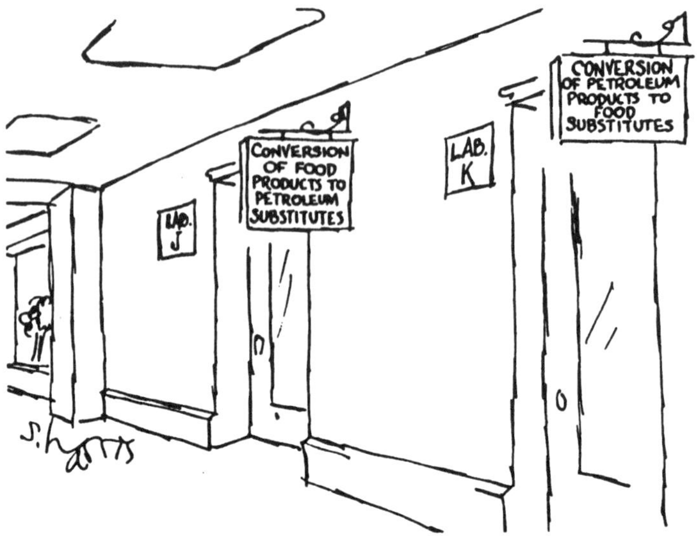
CONVERSION OF FOOD PRODUCTS TO PETROLEUM SUBSTITUTES
LAB. J
LAB. K
CONVERSION OF PETROLEUM PRODUCTS TO FOOD SUBSTITUTES
S. Harris

crease your juicy fruit and salad intake in relation to cooked vegetables, legumes, grains, nuts, and seeds. Whether you acquire your fluids from juicy foods, distilled or purified water, or juices, the effect on your digestion can be similar; and indigestion can occur when fluids are taken in large quantities with drier foods.

Don't eat your meals haphazardly!

It is probably best to ingest your foods beginning with the wettest and ending with the driest. If you think you will need to drink with your meal, drink first. If you are having fruits, have them next, followed by salads, and then other foods. Generally, you will not eat all these things at one meal. However, this method will allow your dehydrated body to absorb fluids quicker without interfering with digestion. Also, the sugar content of fruits usually digests best when eaten before other foods because most other foods take longer to digest and may slow down the absorption of the fruit. This can result in a tendency for fermentation to occur.

Will I still get health benefits from the Natural Hygiene diet if I "fall off the wagon" periodically?
The key word here is *periodically.* Clearly, you do not need to be 100% compliant in order to be healthy. Under normal circumstances, your body is able to compensate to a certain degree for your occasional dietary and lifestyle indiscretions.

But *occasional* indiscretions quickly can become *habitual* ones. Many people find that it is easier for them to develop consistent, long-term, health-promoting behaviors if they eliminate certain old habits entirely, rather than constantly tempting themselves with concentrated sources of sugar, fat, and salt.

Keep in mind that cravings for sugar, fat, and salt helped ensure the survival of our species. In a natural setting, concentrated sources of sugar, fat, and salt are scarce. There are no hamburger bushes or chocolate chip cookie trees. Heated, processed, refined foods do not exist in a natural setting. As a consequence, during our evolutionary history there was no reason to rule out our natural desire for those substances. In fact, in a natural setting, these very drives lead us to fruits, vegetables, and other whole, natural foods.

Today, we have countless varieties of processed foods (each designed to fool your natural instincts) and the desire to eat them is strong. So, you may find that it is easier just to draw the line and not to "occasionally" tease yourself with things that may lead to further consumption.

The longer you practice the Natural Hygiene dietary recommendations, the less interested you will be in unhealthful foods. That is why Hygienic physicians stress the importance of consistency with your diet and lifestyle patterns as part of an overall strategy that will lead to long-term health and happiness.

When I try to give up sugar and caffeine, I experience anxiety, restlessness, nausea, headaches, and irritability. What can I do?

Most people who are addicted to sugar and caffeine are using these as stimulating drugs to try to compensate for fatigue. Although some of these people may seem like they have high-energy, they are usually low-energy, highly stimulated people living on adrenaline. They use sugar or caffeine—or just push themselves physically and mentally—to keep going when their bodies are screaming at them to stop and rest. The net result is that the "fight-or-flight" stress response of the sympathetic nervous system kicks in, for which the main neurotransmitter is adrenaline. Without the "food" drugs, these people feel absolutely wretched from fatigue, not to mention that they cannot function at all if they do not push themselves.

It is extremely difficult to control the cravings for stimulating foods under these conditions because you feel too poorly for your willpower to last very long. Besides, you need energy for willpower. It is not lack of knowledge about what constitutes a healthful diet. Until you deal with the cause of the cravings, which is most likely underlying fatigue, you will not be able to control the eating behavior.

▼ ▼ ▼ ▼ ▼

In the next chapter, you will learn about some of the many Natural Hygiene resources available to you!

12

Natural Hygiene Resources

There are a great many resources available to you as you begin your new, healthier, and happier diet and lifestyle. Take advantage of these very special opportunities to grow in knowledge, experience, and enjoyment.

American Natural Hygiene Society

The American Natural Hygiene Society is the international center for current information and activities in the field of Natural Hygiene. Founded in 1948, the Society is the oldest and largest Natural Hygiene organization in the world, with more than 10,000 members in over seventy countries.

Largest Natural Hygiene organization in the world!

In fulfilling its mission, the Society has created many publications, programs, and services to promote its lifesaving message and to empower people to choose true health independence for themselves and their loved ones.

The Society publishes the award-winning *Health Sci-*

ence magazine; conducts International Natural Living Conferences and Seminars; and publishes and distributes Natural Hygiene books and tapes.

Join the American Natural Hygiene Society today!

Take advantage of the tremendous support system membership in the American Natural Hygiene Society brings.

Great membership benefits!

Membership benefits include:

1. A subscription to the Society's colorful, award-winning membership journal—*Health Science* magazine
2. Discounts on all ANHS Conferences and Seminars
3. Free ANHS book and tape catalog
4. Discounts on all books, audiotapes, and videotapes
5. List of Hygienic physicians who are members of the International Association of Hygienic Physicians
6. Membership card
7. Health alerts on important national issues
8. Free member's decal for your car, and more!

Annual membership dues are $25 in the United States and Canada, $45 in all other countries. To become a member or to get more information, contact:

American Natural Hygiene Society
P.O. Box 30630
Tampa, FL 33630
(813) 855-6607

Health Science magazine

Award ➨ winning magazine!

Health Science is the award-winning membership journal of the American Natural Hygiene Society. Published six times per year, this publication is the only major Natural Hygiene periodical published in the world today, with readers in over seventy countries.

Health Science includes interviews with the world's foremost physicians and teachers of Natural Hygiene, as well as recipes, diet tips, and articles on how to build and maintain exuberant health and a joyful lifestyle.

A one-year subscription to *Health Science* is $25 in the United States and Canada, $45 in all other countries.

To subscribe, contact:

***Health Science* magazine**
P.O. Box 30630
Tampa, FL 33630
(813) 855-6607 *Note: Members of the American Natural Hygiene Society (see opposite page) receive **Health Science** as part of their membership benefits.*

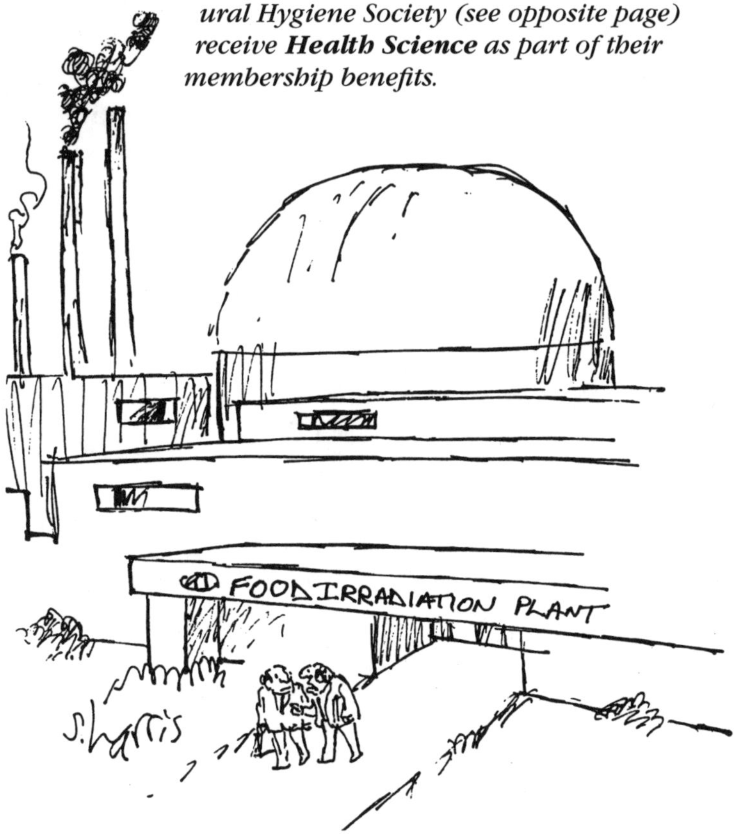

"What we must decide is, if there is a radiation accident which wipes out this entire part of the country, do we pass on the cost to the consumer?"

ANHS on the Internet

Visit the American Natural Hygiene Society's Home Page on the World Wide Web. The Internet is a great way to get information about ANHS, and it is an easy way to introduce people to Natural Hygiene—just give them the ANHS Internet address: www.anhs.org.

Health alerts on important national issues

Members of the American Natural Hygiene Society have been staunch supporters in the fight for safe food and a clean and healthy environment. ANHS fights to keep our organic food supply free from irradiation, genetic engineering, and other potential threats to safety.

To become a member of the Society, see page 127.

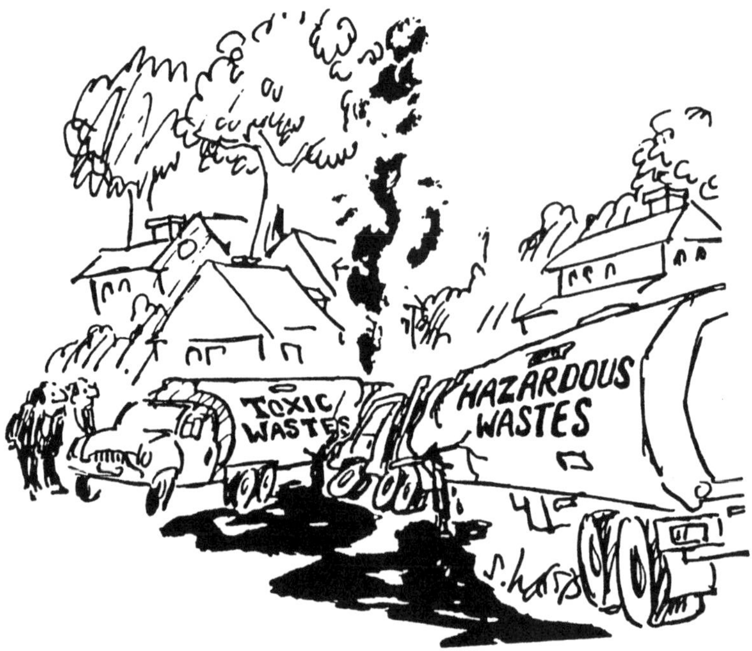

"There goes the neighborhood."

ANHS International Natural Living Conferences and Seminars

Each year, the American Natural Hygiene Society conducts a major International Health Conference. The featured speakers are expert physicians from around the world who specialize in health, nutrition, exercise, prevention, rest, and recovery through natural methods.

← Meet new friends from around the world while learning!

These events have attracted thousands of people through the years. Taped recordings of the lectures and workshops have been distributed to thousands of others. The Society also conducts regional seminars.

For more information, contact the American Natural Hygiene Society. (See page 127.)

Natural Hygiene books and tapes

The American Natural Hygiene Society publishes and distributes thousands of books, audiotapes, and videotapes on the subject of diet and health. The latest, most up-to-date, and accurate information on Natural Hygiene is available on the Society's audiotapes and videotapes. (See page 121.) To get a current catalog, contact the American Natural Hygiene Society. (See page 127.)

Other Natural Hygiene organizations

Australian Natural Hygiene Society
Arcadia Health Center
Cobah Road, Arcadia NSW 2159 AUSTRALIA
61-29-653-1115

British Natural Hygiene Society
Shalimar, Harold Grove
Frinton-On-Sea, Essex
CO13 9BD ENGLAND
441-25-567-2823

Physicians in Natural Hygiene

The International Association of Hygienic Physicians is a professional association for licensed, primary-care physicians (medical doctors, osteopaths, chiropractors, and naturopaths) who provide Hygienic care.

In the case of illness, a person's diet and activities may need to be extensively modified, and he or she may need to be under the supervision of a physician.

You can get a complete list of all of the current members of the International Association of Hygienic Physicians from the American Natural Hygiene Society. (See page 127.)

▼ ▼ ▼ ▼ ▼

In the next chapter, learn how to get the best Natural Hygiene books, audiotapes, and videotapes!

13

Natural Hygiene Books, Audiotapes, and Videotapes

The American Natural Hygiene Society offers a comprehensive collection of books, audiotapes, and videotapes on Natural Hygiene. The most important of them are listed here. To get a complete catalog of the books, audiotapes, and videotapes available, see "Ordering Instructions" at the end of this chapter.

To order Natural Hygiene books and tapes, see p. 124!

The four most important current books on Natural Hygiene are *The Natural Hygiene Handbook, Fasting and Eating For Health, The Health Promoting Cookbook,* and *Dictionary of Natural Foods*.

The Natural Hygiene Handbook

J.M. Lennon and S. Taylor, editors — ***ANHS Book #238***

The best, up-to-date information on Natural Hygiene! This book will answer all of your questions about America's oldest and most revolutionary health system—fasting, diet, and much more. This book should be in the home of everyone who cares about their health. 128 pp.

Fasting and Eating For Health

Joel Fuhrman, M.D. — ***ANHS Book #247***

The most important book of its kind ever! Describes how fasting and aggressive nutritional changes not only can *prevent* disease but can actually *reverse* many serious illnesses. These recommendations for a natural diet are backed by strong scientific documentation. 255 pp.

Best ➨ recipe book!

Health Promoting Cookbook

Alan Goldhamer, D.C. ***ANHS Book #244***

Everything you need to know to adopt or maintain a totally healthful diet is contained in this great new vegan cookbook! The more than 200 recipes are wheat-free and low-fat, and contain no animal products. Added oil, salt, and sugar also are avoided. 186 pp.

Dictionary of Natural Foods

William Esser, N.D. ***ANHS Book #017***

One of the best-selling books on the Natural Hygiene diet. Learn the exact nutrients of all the natural foods—everything you need to know in alphabetical order. Beautiful color photographs, food combining tips, food preparation, exotic fruits, and much more! 166 pp.

To order one of these books, see "Ordering Information" at end of chapter.

Audiotapes

These audiotapes, recorded at annual ANHS International Conferences, provide the most current Natural Hygiene information available!

The best way to get the facts about Natural Hygiene!

Complete Set of ANHS Conference Tapes

Speakers at ANHS International Conferences ***ANHS Audio #(by year)***

Lectures from the annual ANHS International Conferences offer the most comprehensive, up-to-date information on Natural Hygiene available. Topics range from the principles of Natural Hygiene to diet and nutrition, stress management, the role of rest and sleep in the healing process, and how to put your total health program into practice.

Diet and Nutrition *(six tapes)*

Drs. Campbell, Cinque, Goldhamer, Klaper; and V. Moran ***ANHS Audio #9754***

Topics include: Benefits of the Hygienic Diet; Benefits of a Plant-Based, Whole Food Diet; Tailoring the Natural Hygiene Diet to Meet Your Needs; Role of Diet in Health and Disease; Get the Fat Out; and Understanding the Science behind Vegetarian Nutrition.

Women's Health Issues *(six tapes)*

Drs. N. Burton, Fuhrman, Sabatino ***ANHS Audio #9751***

Topics include: Health Concerns of Women; Preventing and Reversing Arthritis and Osteoporosis; Understanding Your Hormones; Successful Weight Management; Women's Health Problems—Breast and Ovarian Cancer; and Facts and Myths about Aging.

Videotapes

Some of the most important lectures at ANHS Conferences

Fabulous Food Festival

Joy Gross ***ANHS Video #304***

The best party food video ever! Entertaining, creative approach to serving natural gourmet party foods. Festive and delicious ideas!

Feeding Healthy Families

Paula Duvall ***ANHS Video #305***

Exciting new ways to prepare meals sure to please your family! Great tips and nutritional information from an experienced gourmet chef!

Understanding the Science behind Vegetarian Nutrition

Michael Klaper, M.D. ***ANHS Video #306***

Up-to-date documentation of why the vegetarian diet works! Get the facts you need to stay healthy. A powerful and entertaining video!

The New Four Food Groups

Neal Barnard, M.D. ***ANHS Video #307***

The New Four Food Groups is the way America will eat in the future! Understand why, from the man who dared to challenge the meat myth!

Health Care of the Future

Joel Fuhrman, M.D. ***ANHS Video #308***

Learn the way of future health care *now* before it's too late! Protect yourself and your family from out-of-date concepts. Offers a powerful look at your real health options!

The Role of Diet in Health and Disease

Alan Goldhamer, D.C. ***ANHS Video #316***

What you eat plays a major role in your overall health. Your eating choices play an important part in how you feel! Learn how to live healthfully and happily from one of the most dynamic speakers in Natural Hygiene.

Successful Weight Management: Why Diets Fail

Frank Sabatino, D.C., Ph.D. ***ANHS Video #320***

Learn how a totally healthful eating program promotes good health and successful weight management. Learn why diets fail and why the body tries to maintain its current weight!

The Benefits of a Plant-Based, Whole-Food Diet

← A must for every student of nutrition!

T. Colin Campbell, Ph.D. ***ANHS Video #323***

This world-renowned researcher presents dramatic, *documented* evidence to support recommendations to eat a plant-based, whole-food diet. An extraordinary look at information you will not see elsewhere.

Classic Historical Books

These classic books were written between 1934 and 1964 by ANHS Co-founder Herbert M. Shelton, D.C., N.D.

Fasting Can Save Your Life

Dr. Herbert M. Shelton ***ANHS Book #182***

Discusses the benefits of fasting in various acute and chronic diseases, including arthritis, colitis, heart disease, and more. It establishes the difference between the popular pseudo-fasts, such as juice or fruit diets, and true fasting, which is abstinence. 195 pp.

Natural Hygiene: The Pristine Way of Life

Dr. Herbert M. Shelton ***ANHS Book #219***

Considered by many to have been the most important book on Natural Hygiene ever written! Describes the total Natural Hygiene system as seen from the author's many decades of experience. 640 pp.

The Science and Fine Art of Food and Nutrition

Dr. Herbert M. Shelton ***ANHS Book #007***

Discusses our nutritional needs; what nutrition is; and what, when, and how to eat. It examines fruitarianism, vegetarianism, food combining, raw foods, the feeding of children, and more. 591 pp.

Ordering Information

How to order! ➡

To order ANHS books, audiotapes, or videotapes with your VISA or MasterCard, please call (813) 855-6607, or fax (813) 855-8052, or E-mail anhs@anhs.org. Ordering hours are: 10am–4pm Mon.–Fri. Or write for a catalog: ANHS, P.O. Box 30630, Tampa, FL 33630.

▼ ▼ ▼ ▼ ▼

In the next chapter, you will learn how to become an American Natural Hygiene Society member!

14

Becoming an ANHS Member

Now that you have learned about the benefits of the Natural Hygiene diet, we hope that you will want to become a member of the American Natural Hygiene Society (ANHS). In addition to all of the other benefits you will receive, ANHS membership can be a tremendous support system for you.

ANHS is the international center for current information and activities in the field of Natural Hygiene. Founded in 1948, the Society is the oldest and largest Natural Hygiene organization in the world, with more than 10,000 members in over seventy countries.

By becoming an ANHS member, you create a powerful partnership that will bring tremendous rewards. You will *receive* many tangible benefits—a subscription to the award-winning *Health Science* magazine; discounts on all ANHS Conferences and Seminars; discounts on Natural Hygiene books, audiotapes, and videotapes; ongoing updates about critical health issues, such as food irradiation and important legislation; and much more!

← ***Valuable benefits!***

Your ➡ support makes a big difference!

By being an ANHS member, you also *give* a tremendous gift. Your ongoing membership helps ANHS spread the lifesaving message of Natural Hygiene to people around the world. The support of knowledgeable, caring people like you can mean the difference between life and death for people who are suffering needlessly for lack of information.

Join the American Natural Hygiene Society today!

Take advantage of the tremendous support system that membership in the Society brings.

Membership benefits include:

1. A subscription to the Society's colorful, award-winning membership journal—*Health Science* magazine
2. Discounts on all ANHS Conferences and Seminars
3. Free ANHS book and tape catalog
4. Discounts on all books, audiotapes, and videotapes
5. List of Hygienic physicians who are members of the International Association of Hygienic Physicians
6. Health alerts on important national issues
7. Membership card
8. Free member's decal for your car, and more!

Annual membership dues are only $25 in the United States and Canada, $45 in all other countries. To become a member or to get more information, contact:

American Natural Hygiene Society
P.O. Box 30630
Tampa, FL 33630
(813) 855-6607 (Voice)
(813) 855-8052 (Fax)
www.anhs.org
anhs@anhs.org (E-mail)